Waist Away

*How I lost 70 Pounds
In 7 Months Without
Drugs or Surgery*

3rd Edition

Dr. John Reizer

Waist Away

*How I lost 70 Pounds
In 7 Months Without
Drugs or Surgery*

3rd Edition

By

Dr. John Reizer

Dr. John Reizer

Contents

Dr. John Reizer

About The Author

Dr. John Reizer is a 1986 magna cum laude graduate of Sherman College of Straight Chiropractic. Born in Lakewood, New Jersey in 1963, he returned home to his native state after graduating from college and operated two successful chiropractic offices for 12 years. In 1998, Dr. Reizer returned to Sherman College and served as a member of the teaching faculty until January, 2010. He currently operates a private practice in Boiling Springs, SC. More information is available at www.johnreizer.com.

Dr. John Reizer

Disclaimer

The information contained within this book has not been evaluated by the FDA. The information is for educational purposes only and is not intended to diagnose, treat, cure, or prevent any disease!

Prior to beginning any diet or exercise program, including a walking routine, you should consult a physician to make sure that you are physically capable of safely taking part in such a program.

In addition, the information that has been written in this book is based upon the opinions of Dr. John Reizer. The information is not intended to replace a professional relationship between a patient and a healthcare specialist nor is it intended as medical advice. This information is provided solely for the purpose of sharing knowledge derived from the experience of Dr. John Reizer. Dr. Reizer strongly encourages readers to make healthcare decisions based upon their own independent research.

Dr. John Reizer

Introduction

My name is John Reizer and this is a true account of how I lost a total of seventy pounds in a period of seven months. In January of 2007, I decided to weigh myself on a bathroom scale and instantly confirmed what I had suspected for quite a lengthy period of time; I was extremely overweight! I hadn't stepped on a scale in about two years and I knew that I was out of shape, but I had no idea just how heavy and how out of shape I had become.

At the age of 44, I decided that it was finally time to view the damage and so after some moments of quiet contemplation, I convinced myself that I needed to step on that bathroom scale. As the numbers flickered to life, they gradually settled at the ridiculous weight of 245 pounds. I instantly became very depressed. Those feelings of depression were soon replaced by the feelings of anger and later by fear. I was disgusted, depressed, and scared all at once.

Up to that point in time, it had been very easy for me to rationalize, in my own mind, about being comfortable with my weight. It's quite amazing how a person can, over a period of time, continue to gain weight and, for the most part, be unaware of the actual accumulation of extra pounds on his or her body. In some respects it is analogous to a snow storm. You do not hear the snow flakes as they come floating down from the clouds above. The next morning when you look out your front window you see that the storm delivered several feet of snow on the ground and you are left with quite a mess. The same can be said about gaining weight as the process seems quite innocuous as it is taking place, but eventually it leaves you with a heck of a problem over time.

Looking back at my own situation, it became obvious to me that I had been living in a constant state of denial for a number of years. A blizzard had taken place inside of me and now, as I looked at myself in the mirror, I finally realized that I had become trapped in a body that was 70 pounds too heavy.

My professional background as a healthcare provider immediately sent warning signals to my educated mind. I knew that I had to weather this storm and get my problem under control fast. I remember quite vividly coming out to the living room to talk with my wife about my new found discovery. I told her, with a great amount of emotion in my voice, *I was a fat slob.* She began laughing. She and I had both known for a couple of years that I had a serious weight problem. It had struck her funny when I came out of the bathroom and declared myself fat. We both laughed for a few moments and then discussed my dilemma in a more serious manner.

Over the past couple of years my weight gain had caused me to develop a problem with snoring. My poor wife could not even sleep in the same room with me because my snoring kept her up the entire night. This snoring issue became the source of many heated arguments between us. On numerous occasions I can remember instructing her not to keep waking me from a deep sleep. I reasoned with her that at least one of us should be able to get some rest. On yet another occasion, I went on a business trip with my brother to Sacramento, California where we shared a hotel room. The initial morning after we slept in that hotel room my brother presented me with a tape recording which he had made of me snoring during the previous night. He commented that he had never heard anyone snore as loud as I had. When I listened to the recording, I could not believe my ears. I had no idea just how much my problem had progressed.

Another problem I had developed over the past couple of years was a constant lack of energy. It seemed as though I was always tired. This lack of energy was quite annoying. I wanted to be more physically active, but it seemed that a nap or sitting in front of the television was a more attractive choice for me. I was also beginning to experience episodes of shortness of breath when I would have to walk up a hill or climb a set of stairs. This, more than any other symptomatic change in my life, began to grab my attention and ultimately initiated the process of waking me up from the deep coma like trance I had been stuck in.

For a good portion of my life I had been in very good physical shape. In my high school years I excelled in organized sports such as baseball and football. During my years in college, and even after I graduated from chiropractic college, I remained very active, running and exercising at a fitness center several times a week. Throughout my 20's and well into my 30's, I did a tremendous amount of running as well. I would often run about 20 – 30 miles a week on an indoor track. I usually maintained a weight right around 175 pounds during those years. I am approximately 5' 11 inches tall and I have always believed that I looked and felt my best at this weight.

In January, 2007 I was far away from looking and feeling good. I was also far away from my optimum weight of 175 pounds. During the past 8 years I had lived a more sedentary and stressful lifestyle than ever before. My employment as an assistant professor at a chiropractic college in those years had been quite enjoyable to me, but the position also brought a great deal of stress into my life.

The demands of academia, as well as adapting to a new lifestyle that came along with the birth of my beautiful daughter in 2001, presented me with a number of stresses that I had not previously experienced. I also authored 5 books over a 4 year span of time. My focus had been centered on a word processor and not on an indoor track where I would have been dedicated to a workout program. When you regularly engage in *brain work,* you often feel like you are working hard, but in a physical sense you are hardly working. I did not get fat and out of shape in one or two weeks. It took a major commitment to living a completely sedentary lifestyle to accomplish the amount of weight gain that I had achieved.

The simple facts were that I was 70 pounds over weight; I had little or no energy; I was regularly experiencing episodes of shortness of breath when taking part in light exercise, and I was very much terrified about my predicament. I really had no idea what to do to get myself out of this situation. I was scared to admit to anyone that I had a serious problem. In January, 2007, I believed that I needed the services of a trained professional in order to help me out of my living hell. I knew that if I continued with my current lifestyle that I probably would not live for very long.

My healthcare training as a licensed doctor of chiropractic made it clear to me that I was probably facing a lifetime of weight related health disorders such as diabetes, cardiovascular problems, autoimmune challenges, and increased pressure on my skeletal system, which also increased my chances of developing osteoarthritis throughout most of the bony joints in my body. I knew there were a multitude of other potential health problems that I would quite possibly encounter if I actually lived long enough. Basically, the entire quality of my life would become substandard if I did not solve this problem. One way or another, I had to save my life and I felt that I had to take action immediately.

What you are about to read is the blue print that saved my life. I am writing about my experience because I believe there are many people living in the United States that might be able to benefit from my story. I know there are people out there that want to lose weight; that want to be more physically active, and that want to have more energy than they currently possess. I changed my life in just 7 months and so can you. The people that know me continue to be amazed at the physical changes I have made in just a relatively short period of time. At the time of this writing, I am regularly receiving requests from students, colleagues, and friends for information on how they can *"Waist Away"* and duplicate the dramatic weight loss results which I have achieved. These people are absolutely amazed that I was able to pull off such a major accomplishment without utilizing any type of arduous exercise program, expensive gym equipment, prepackaged food plans, dangerous drugs or surgical procedures. I was also able to eat a healthy diet, and I never once starved or deprived myself of any valuable nutritional requirements.

I encourage you to read this book in its entirety. It is my hope that the people who are facing what I once faced will be able to help themselves by reading about my own personal experience.

Whenever I am able to educate myself with valuable information about healthcare concepts, I feel it is important for me to share the material with others. Because I wear the title doctor, *(the Latin translation for the word doctor is teacher)* I have an even larger obligation than the average person to follow through on revealing important information about health related topics to laypersons. I truly believe that the acquisition and delivery of healthcare knowledge, through the reading and writing of books, is an essential component in keeping the members of our society at an optimal level of health. This is my story.

John L. Reizer, D.C.
Chiropractor

The Risks Associated With Being Overweight

During the years that I studied to become a chiropractor, I had been exposed to a fair amount of information about health through good nutrition. My formal education, which included 4 years of chiropractic college, provided me with various courses in physiology, biochemistry, and nutrition. I was aware of the inherent risks associated with being overweight, and in my own case I knew that I had fallen into a category that labeled me as being obese.

According to most experts in the field of nutrition, I was considered an obese person for my height and weight. The healthcare industry utilizes two formulas to categorize a person's status in regards to being overweight or obese. The first formula is known as the *Body Mass Index* (BMI) which is basically a fancy title for assessing a person's weight in relationship to his or her height.

(Please refer to the chart below.)

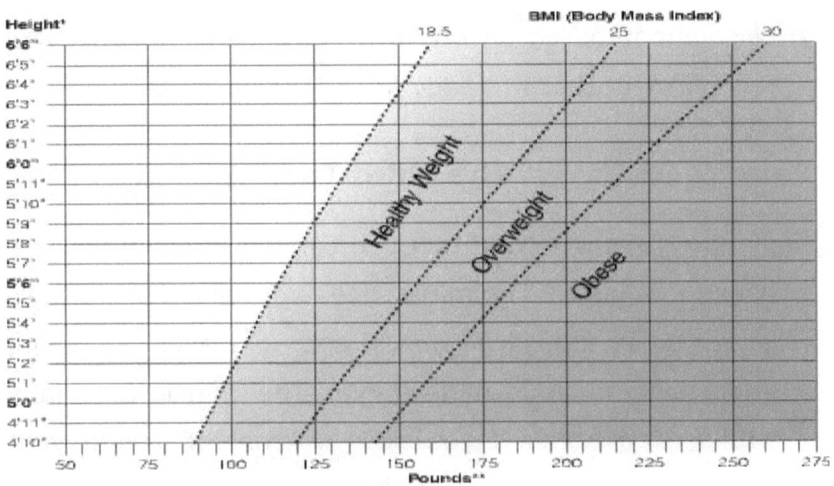

Find your weight on the bottom of the graph. Go straight up from that point until you come to the line that matches your height. Then look to find your weight group. The higher your BMI is over 25, the greater chance you may have of developing health problems.

Source – WIN: U.S. Department of Health and Human Services

The other tool that is commonly utilized to categorize people as being overweight or obese is measuring the circumference of the waist with a tape measure. A measurement greater than 35 inches for a woman or 40 inches for a man sends out warning signals to healthcare experts. So basically if you have a BMI that is 25 or higher, or a waist circumference measurement that is greater than 35 inches for a female, and greater than 40 inches for a male, you are either overweight or obese and you are a prime candidate for various diseases. I did some quick calculations based on my own body measurements and reconfirmed what I already knew—I was obese!

The Third Tool

There is a third tool you can use to tell if you are obese – a mirror. The mirror does not tell a lie. A picture is worth a thousand words and it leaves a lasting impression in your mind's eye. The mirror technique works even better if you pose in front of it with your clothes off. I found this method motivated me the most in regards to convincing me that I had a serious problem.

More Determined Than Ever

At the age of 44 I was classified as an obese person. I was writing bestselling books on the subject of chiropractic and I was deeply involved in the process of educating future doctors while simultaneously giving out advice to my patients in a private practice setting. I thought to myself, *why would anyone want to take healthcare advice from someone who was obese and out of shape?* I then asked myself an even more painful question. *Would I take healthcare advice from someone who looked like me?* After thinking the question over for a few seconds, the answer I came up with was – absolutely not.

As my BMI increased, my self esteem began to shrink. I was definitely not feeling very good about me at this point. After reviewing all of this information in my mind, I knew deep down inside that I had absolutely reached a critical point in my life and it was time to take immediate action. I was more determined than ever to carry out my plan. I could be a very disciplined and determined person if I put my mind on something. I felt, for the first time in many years, I had the focus and the proper attitude to get my weight problem corrected permanently. If I failed to correct my problem I was very aware of the health risks that I would have to face.

Assessing the Risks of Obesity

As I stated in the introduction of this book, the risks associated with obesity are numerous. *Osteo Arthritis,* which is caused from the wear and tear of the body's bony joints, is a big problem and it is definitely linked to increased weight gain. Excessive weight on the skeletal system causes the joints in the body to become misaligned from one another or to shift slightly and this in turn causes the body to cement the bones in place by placing calcium deposits around the various joints involved. This is an attempt by the body to try and stabilize an already unstable situation. *Osteoarthritis* is a defense mechanism employed by the body and the condition can be very painful while causing massive destruction to the knees, hip joints and the spinal column. Keep in mind that the spinal column protects the spinal cord which happens to be the "life line" of the entire human body.

Hypertension (High Blood Pressure) is another risk associated with being overweight. *Hypertension* can place a tremendous strain on the entire cardiovascular system and it can eventually lead to heart disease and strokes. Many studies have been conducted, over the years, and they demonstrate that just a minimal degree of weight loss can impact a person's blood pressure in a positive way.

Along with being fat comes the chance of developing problems with the liver and the gallbladder. Obesity eventually causes these organs to have increased work loads, and over time pathologies will surface. Increased amounts of fat deposits near or around the liver can cause inflammation and a lack of vascular supply to the organ. A lack of blood supply can cause necrotic changes to take place and then scar tissue forms in the liver which ultimately can lead to a non functional organ.

In the case of the gallbladder, it is common to see an increase in gall stone formation in those people who are overweight. It is not completely understood why this happens but the fact that it does occur is reason enough to take the extra pounds off your body.

Another serious condition which develops in people who are obese is the condition known as *Sleep Apnea*. *Sleep Apnea* occurs when there are too many fat cells around the neck and throat region. The fat cells place an unusual amount of pressure in the person's airway when he or she is sleeping or lying down. This obstruction will often cause the person to snore very loud and in some cases the individual will stop breathing completely and will wake up gasping for air. Over an extended period of time, *Sleep Apnea* can cause *pulmonary hypertension* which is usually a fatal condition.

Many cancers are also linked to obesity. Although the exact mechanisms that trigger the various forms of cancer are not really understood, it is now widely accepted by most conventional thinking healthcare specialists that the risk of cancer in a person can be dramatically reduced if the individual can maintain a proper diet and commit to a sensible weight loss campaign.

The chance of developing *diabetes* also increases dramatically for those people who are obese or overweight. *Diabetes* can affect the circulatory system, promote vision problems, initiate nervous system disorders and most importantly is a major cause of death in the United States. Once again, a person who faces this type of risk can reduce his or her chance of developing the disease just by losing some extra pounds.

The health risks that were associated with my body shape and size had been laid out very clearly for me to see. I knew that I had to set some specific goals and get the logistics for accomplishing this monumental task worked out. It was very early in January, 2007 and I was damned determined that by the end of August, 2007 I was going to be seventy pounds lighter.

I want my readers to remember that I never used shakes, diet pills, fad diets, prepackaged meals, expensive gym memberships, or the services of a personal fitness trainer. This is the true story of how I accomplished an almost impossible task in a seven month period of time.

Setting My Goals

Setting my personal goals and making them realistic enough so that I could attain them in a reasonable amount of time would ultimately help to facilitate the process of returning me to my target weight of 175 pounds.

There is a definite methodology to consider when setting goals. It was not something that I wanted to rush into blindly without carefully planning. I was serious about being successful in this particular area of my life and I knew that it was essential that I took the time to carefully think about what I really wanted to accomplish.

I knew that visualization techniques were extremely useful when creating goals. If you cannot visualize an objective you are trying to accomplish, it is highly unlikely that you will be able to succeed in your venture. Once I was able to visualize what I wanted to accomplish, I needed to take a mental snap shot of that image. It was important that I captured, in my mind's eye, the essence of that mental image and that I never forgot it.

Next, I needed to write down on a piece of paper the types of personal goals I wanted to accomplish. I began by writing a rough draft of my goals into a few simple sentences. Writing the information on paper helped me to make the intangible, tangible. This was a crucial step in the goal setting process because it took the visual picture, which I created, and transformed it directly into my total perceived reality.

When I began writing my personal weight loss goals, it was important for me to remember that I had to construct them in a realistic manner. I also needed to avoid making them too large. Really big goals needed to be reduced to smaller objectives. This would prevent me from becoming overwhelmed by the size of a particular task. I had to keep in mind that large or small unrealistic goals could lead me into a corner filled with frustration which would ultimately prevent me from becoming successful in accomplishing my objectives.

I kept my goals very specific. I did not want to write down a bunch of objectives that were too general or vague. This could lead to problems later on. It was also important to make my goals very private and applicable to only one person – me! I would not, under any circumstances, allow friends or family members to help me author these weight loss objectives. I was the person who had taken the mental snapshot of where I wanted to be and therefore I had to be the only person writing down all of the pertinent information.

I believed that it was extremely important for me to construct various schedules for the goals I would be setting along with specific dates that I expected to attain them. Goals that are set without immediate timetables are difficult to achieve. By attaching schedules to my goals, I would be able to pace myself and I could very easily track the level of my progress over time. A schedule also allowed me the flexibility to modify a specific goal should this become necessary.

The next step in this process was for me to prioritize my goals. This would help me to classify and separate my primary objectives from the far less important objectives. I felt this could also be a big help in keeping me focused, on the bigger picture, while simultaneously allowing me to remain realistic in my approach so that I could take care of any housekeeping that needed to be dealt with.

Now that I had my *preliminary goals* prioritized into clear, specific, personalized objectives, I wanted to assess whether or not any modifications needed to be made at this point. Did my written goals represent the visual image that I previously constructed? If the written and the visual components matched, I was in good shape. If the written and visual components were not congruent, I would definitely need to modify the written information so that it matched the original visual snapshot in my mind. I needed to take my *preliminary goals* and adjust them accordingly. In either scenario, the written and visual components had to mirror one another. Once this was achieved, I then referred to my *preliminary goals* as my *adjusted goals*.

Once my *adjusted goals* had been finalized, I wanted to identify any barriers or possible obstacles that might prevent me from accomplishing what I had placed on paper. In my own view, the obstacles I might theoretically encounter were the items in my life that I could not afford to focus on. I knew that if I took my eyes off the major goal I was shooting for, I would see nothing but the various obstacles that were standing in my way. Examples of such obstacles might be laziness or procrastination, as well as a multitude of other excuses that could work their way into the equation. I knew that in certain instances people sometimes constructed such barriers because they were afraid of being successful at something. Once these individuals became cognizant of what they were actually doing, they were often more productive and able to reposition their line of vision back in the direction of the original objective, and the obstacles suddenly and miraculously vanished. I made a personal choice not to focus on the obstacles but rather to focus exclusively on my goals.

I had now created a written blue print which would help to ensure my future success. It was going to be imperative that I stayed loyal to my cause. It was one thing to write down a game plan, and quite another thing to execute the plan to a level that was necessary to win the game.

It would be important for me to periodically track the level of my progress as well as to review the goals I had written down. I also needed to continue to try and visualize the results I was trying to achieve on a regular basis.

I have prepared worksheets on the next few pages of this book that demonstrate the process I utilized in setting up my own written goals. I would suggest to readers that you carefully study the data I created so that you can utilize a similar approach when you begin to set your own weight loss goals.

After you design your own worksheets and fill in the information, you should consider constructing some charts which will help you track your progress over time. The use of charts will be helpful in keeping you focused and excited about accomplishing the various personal objectives you are working toward. Measuring your progress along with repetitiously reviewing your goals on a daily basis will allow you to form positive habits that will greatly increase your chances of being successful in completing your own weight loss objectives.

Written Goals Worksheet

1. Write down in a few sentences the goals that you have previously visualized.

I would like to see myself at a healthy weight of 175 pounds. I see myself reaching my objective by eating healthy foods, controlling my portion sizes and by incorporating regular intervals of exercise within my daily lifestyle.

2. Each major goal should then be broken down into smaller goals or objectives.

a) **I have a target weight of 175 pounds.**

b) **I will consume healthy foods & portions.**

c) **I will exercise on a daily basis.**

Written Goals Worksheet

3. Write down an estimated date of completion for each of the smaller goals that you listed.

        a) **8/31/07**

        b) **1/10/07**

        c) **1/10/07**

4. Prioritize the smaller goals that you have listed.

        1) **I will consume healthy foods & portions.**

        2) **I will exercise on a daily basis.**

        3) **I have a target weight of 175 pounds.**

Written Goals Worksheet

5. Do the preliminary, prioritized, smaller goals match or represent the visual image you have made in your mind?

YES!

6. If the answer to question number five is "YES," you should proceed to item number eight on this worksheet. If the answer to item number five is "NO," you should adjust your preliminary goals in the spaces provided in item number seven.

7. Rewrite your smaller goals so that they are congruent with the visual image you constructed prior to writing the original sentences on this worksheet.

1) **Not Applicable**

2) **Not Applicable**

3) **Not Applicable**

Written Goals Worksheet

8. List your finalized "Adjusted Goals" which match your mental snapshot.

    1) **I will consume only healthy foods.**

    2) **I will exercise on a daily basis.**

    3) **I will have a target weight of 175 pounds.**

9. List possible barriers/obstacles that might prevent you from reaching your "Adjusted Goals."

    1. Lack of Family Support

    2. Laziness

    3. Lack of perceived progress

Sample Charts That I Constructed

Projected Weekly Walk Schedule

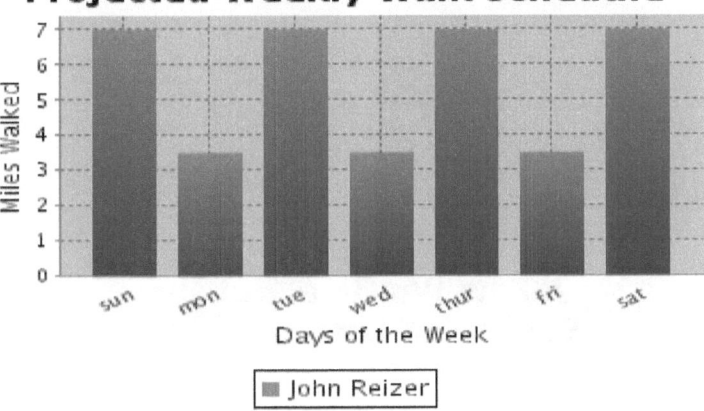

Projected Weight Loss

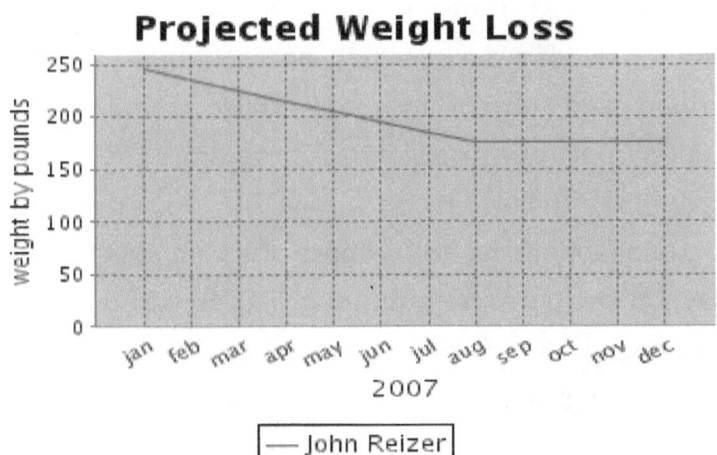

A Few Words about the
Subject of Losing Weight

I was ready to dive head first into my program. I had written my goals and produced some impressive looking charts that I propped up on a desk in my home office. My next order of business was to take the knowledge I had accumulated as a chiropractor about nutrition and physiology, and utilize some of that material in my own "waist away" program.

For those readers who are not very knowledgeable about the subject of losing weight, I will devote this chapter to educating you about some basic information.

A long time ago when you were enrolled in a public or private school, you probably learned in a science course the definition of a calorie. A calorie is defined by the *Oxford Mini Reference Dictionary* as *"a unit of the energy—producing value of food."* The United States Department of Health and Human Services defines a calorie in its excellent publication *"A Healthier You"* in the following way. *"A calorie is the amount of heat needed to raise the temperature of a liter of water 1 degree."* I'm sure those two definitions have absolutely clarified for readers what a calorie is and what it represents.

In a nutshell, a calorie (kilocalorie when pertaining to food) represents potential energy for the human body. When you eat a piece of food, it contains a number of kilocalories that represent potential energy for your body. A kilocalorie might be utilized by your body to perform certain tasks in the present or it can be stored as fat for future use. In either scenario, it is a unit of energy that fuels the physiological processes occurring inside all of us.

The compounds which produce energy (kilocalories) and are contained in all foods are broken down into three categories known as carbohydrates, proteins, and fats. When you consume 1 gram of protein or carbohydrate, you have offered your body four kilocalories of potential energy. When you consume 1 gram of fat, you have offered your body 9 kilocalories of potential energy. It therefore takes the body longer to burn off the fuel from one gram of fat consumption than it does from one gram of protein or carbohydrate consumption. Fats are higher in their kilocalorie values than proteins and carbohydrates.

In order for people to remain healthy, it is necessary for them to consume a certain amount of carbohydrates, fats, & proteins on a daily basis. Most health experts have stated that men and women should have a daily diet that contains percentages somewhere in the range of 45-65% carbohydrates, 20-35% fats, and 10-35% proteins. Every person's physiological makeup is somewhat unique and sometimes, depending on the health requirements of various people, the percentages of these energy producing compounds they will need to consume will vary considerably.

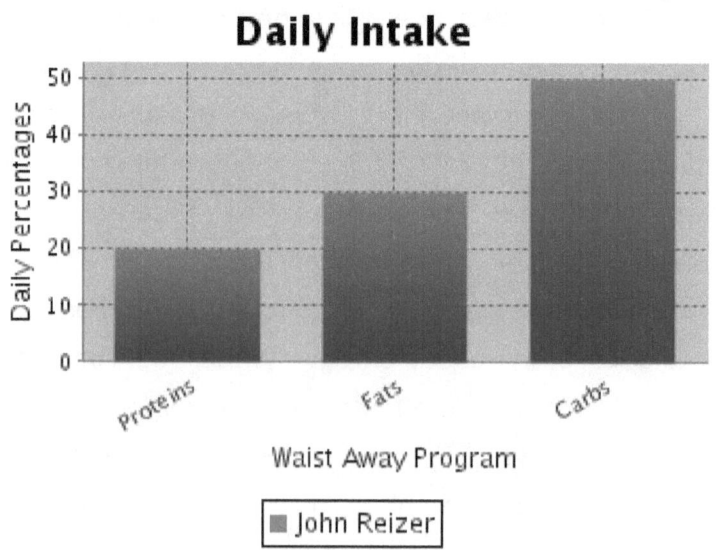

In creating my own diet plan, I decided to consume on a daily basis approximately 50 percent carbohydrates, 30% fats and 20% proteins. If, for example, I consumed 1,800 kilocalories on a given day, I would have consumed those calories by eating the percentages indicated above.

Adding & Losing Pounds

You should now have a basic understanding of what a calorie is. You should also be able to comprehend the concept that the calories which you consume on a daily basis are received through the consumption of compounds known as carbohydrates, proteins, and fats.

I can now explain to you how you can gain or lose weight over time. In order to gain or lose one pound, you have to either have an excess or deficit of 3500 kilocalories from your daily dietary intake. It does not matter how long this process takes. The only requirement for this to occur is that a certain number of kilocalories need to be taken in and a certain number of kilocalories need to be burned by your body's metabolism.

Metabolism

The metabolism is the process in which the body is utilizing the kilocalories inside of you as a source of fuel in order to maintain life. When you exercise, your body's metabolism will increase the rate in which it burns up the body's fuel (kilocalories). Even after you finish an exercise routine, the body's metabolic rate remains elevated for a substantial period of time which causes the body to continue to burn its fuel at a faster rate. The metabolism is always at work, burning kilocalories in order to keep the body functioning in a healthy manner. When you are sitting down watching television or sleeping in bed during the middle of the night, your metabolism is still burning kilocalories. Many people fail to realize that the body constantly requires fuel to maintain life.

Body Composition

The composition of a person's body has a lot to do with how efficiently his or her metabolism burns calories. People that have more body fat than muscle will generally have a slower metabolism. These people will burn calories at a much slower rate. People that have more body muscle than fat will generally have a faster metabolism, and will burn calories at a faster rate. It is because of these factors that many people will work out with weights to create more muscle mass on their bodies. As the muscle mass on a given individual increases through weight training, the person's ability to burn its fuel more efficiently will also increase.

As human beings grow older, they tend to use their muscles less and we begin to experience a general loss of muscle mass. As this process unfolds, it is very common to see elderly people begin to have a slower rate of metabolism. As a person's metabolism slows down, he or she will usually experience some degree of weight gain over time.

Other components of body composition, such as the size and thickness of the skeletal system, might also influence a person's metabolism. Many scientists continue to speculate that there are genetic considerations that have a great influence on the body's rate of metabolism as well.

Gradual Changes in Weight

Let us pretend that you have a diet that allows you to consume on a daily basis 116 more kilocalories than you are burning up through the body's metabolism. At the end of one month you will have an excess of approximately 3,500 kilocalories which will place one additional pound of weight on your body. This might seem like a very insignificant amount of kilocalories, but at the end of a single year you would have added approximately twelve pounds to your body. The same process obviously works in reverse. If you are eating a diet that causes you to have a 116 kilocalorie deficit everyday, you are going to see a monthly weight loss of

41

about one pound. At the end of the year you would remove twelve pounds from your body. This is foolproof science and not based on a theory or some type of conjecture. It is a reproducible part of human physiology, and it will work everyday of the year, as long as you are alive.

Gimmicks & Fad Diets

If something sounds too good to be true then you should probably avoid the offer in question. Chances are quite good that your gut feeling will probably turn out to be correct. In other words, there are no short cuts in life and the same can be said when it comes to the subjects of weight loss and weight gain. So many people in the United States are overweight or obese. Many of these people are desperate to try and find a way out of their situation, and they will try anything that is rumored to work.

There are loads of "fad diets" circulating on the Internet, as well as other information outlets that people regularly access. I was not in the mood to try short cuts that were going to give me quick results very early in my program and would then lead to my failure at a later date. I wanted to construct a program that was going to give me ironclad, positive results. I certainly was not going to drink a vanilla milk shake for breakfast and lunch and then eat one meal for supper. I knew that a plan like that I would toss in the garbage after a couple of weeks. I needed something I could embrace today, tomorrow, next week, and ultimately for the remainder of my life. Milk Shakes were certainly not the answer for me.

Another popular approach I wanted no part of was the very drastic reduction of carbohydrates from my diet for a number of weeks or months. Whenever you deprive your body of essential components of nutrition, something usually suffers down the road. I wanted to make myself lighter and healthier at the same time. Cutting out carbohydrates, proteins, or fats from my daily intake of food would, in my opinion, create a great amount of stress on my already stressed out body.

Several patients that I had been taking care of in my private practice had recently enlisted the services of a popular company on television that would sell its clients prepackaged meals. These products actually worked, and the people consuming the meals were able to lose various amounts of weight after following the pre-designed programs for several months. The problem with a prepackaged meal plan is that it can be extremely expensive and the consumer is not becoming educated about how to prepare his or her own menu. In a prepackaged system, you are at the complete mercy of the company preparing your meals. I believe this approach might work very well with certain people, but it would not be something I would be interested in. I would want to know how to prepare the meals and I would also want to know that I could function in a successful manner if the company suddenly went out of business.

Changing My Lifestyle

If I really wanted to become successful at accomplishing the goals I had previously set, I was going to have to change my lifestyle. Fad diets may work initially, but over the span of several months the results are less impressive. If you interview many of the people who have tried these weight loss schemes, they will tell you that they were miserable while on the diets and, in many cases, they gained back all of the weight they had initially lost. In some cases they gained all of their weight back and gained additional weight as well.

I knew that any weight loss program that was going to work for me would have to be based on consuming healthy foods, monitoring my daily caloric intake, and incorporating a healthy level of daily exercise into my life. This would have to be my new lifestyle plan and there was absolutely no short cut or alternative way to go about accomplishing my ultimate goal.

Is It Safe to Begin My Program?

Before you begin any exercise routine or engage in any type of weight loss program, I highly recommend you make an appointment with a medical doctor and get a physical evaluation. I would also get some blood work processed by a lab, and I would discuss with my healthcare professional the goals that you have set and will be trying to attain. I think it is important to know if it is safe for you to proceed with a particular program. You might discover, through a medical evaluation, that there are health challenges you currently have which might make it dangerous for you to proceed with your weight loss plan. It is better to learn about this type of a problem before you begin working out as opposed to learning about a problem after it has caused you a major health dilemma.

The second thing you should do before you begin your diet and exercise program is to make an appointment with a qualified doctor of chiropractic to have the integrity of your spinal column's alignment assessed. Many people in the United States have never visited a chiropractor before. Their understanding about what regular chiropractic care can do to improve their health is very different from the understanding chiropractic patients have about the same subject matter.

The History of Chiropractic

The word chiropractic comes from the two Greek words *cheiro* and *praktos* which translated into English means the practice done with the hands. Throughout the history of this planet, human beings have been experimenting with the art of spinal adjusting. There are many references found in ancient records giving accounts of this type of health methodology, which was used in an effort to promote healing in the sick and elderly.

Evidence of spinal adjusting has been found in documents that date back to ancient civilizations such as those found in China, Egypt, and Greece. This information was passed on in secret writings and eventually found its way to the 19th century, where health practitioners discovered the same important connections between the nervous system, spinal integrity, and general health disorders.

Later on, an interest in spinal adjustments developed in many additional areas of the world including America. Medical doctors began to regularly utilize such techniques on patients.

In 1895, Daniel David Palmer, a magnetic healer in Davenport, Iowa who was very knowledgeable in human anatomy and physiology, delivered the first modern day chiropractic adjustment to a deaf janitor named Harvey Lillard. The adjustment became famous as Mr. Lillard regained most of his hearing. At first, Palmer thought that he had accidentally stumbled on a cure for deafness. This however, he found not to be the case as other patients with deafness did not respond in the same way as Mr. Lillard. Although this was somewhat frustrating, Palmer was not completely discouraged because in his failure to find a cure for deafness, he began to notice other physiological problems begin to improve in patients to whom he was administering chiropractic adjustments.

Palmer began to slowly make the connections that vertebrae which were out of their proper alignment were not causing a specific malady in the body, but instead were interfering with the body's ability to process information from the brain. The brain was sending the proper messages for the body to be healthy.

The misalignments in the spinal column were distorting these messages and the chemistry of the body began to make mistakes which eventually caused a decline in the health of that person. Palmer rationalized that a correction of these spinal misalignments would restore proper communication between brain and body, thus chemistry in the individual would balance out naturally.

Dr. Palmer started his own chiropractic school in Davenport. Later, his son B.J. Palmer would take over the school and would oversee the formation of the Palmer College of Chiropractic. B.J. Palmer would go on to perform extensive research in the field of chiropractic and would later author numerous articles and books about the science of chiropractic. He was also the chiropractor who developed many of the spinal analysis and adjusting techniques which are still, for the most part, utilized today.

The Chiropractic Objective

The practice objective of chiropractic is really simple to understand. It is a healthcare profession that begins with a very logical premise that human beings have an inborn ability to maintain their health naturally. Chiropractic teaches that the inborn intelligence that runs the body is expressed through the nervous system and that regular uninhibited functioning of the nervous system is necessary for a proper state of health to flourish.

Doctors of chiropractic periodically examine the spine for the purpose of evaluating spinal alignment. Spinal bones (vertebrae) that lose their proper anatomical alignment in relationship to other spinal segments can place pressure on portions of the central and peripheral nervous system. Interference to the human nervous system can disrupt the various physiological processes that are necessary to maintain life.

Chiropractors should be recognized as important members of any community's healthcare team because their professional practice objective of locating, analyzing, and correcting vertebral subluxations contributes dramatically to the overall level of health of citizens throughout the world.

The nervous system coordinates many physiological activities in a human being including immune system functions and proper body metabolism. If patients become compromised and their immune systems are engaged in fighting off various diseases, they are going to have a much better chance of defeating each disease they encounter if their nervous systems are working without disruptions coming from misaligned spinal bones (subluxations).

People who are contemplating the addition of a new workout schedule into their lives will definitely want to maintain proper spinal alignment and an efficient running nervous system. This will help to ensure that your metabolic rate will operate at a maximum level of efficiency.

As I prepared to commence my *waist away* program, I received a medical evaluation and stepped up the level of chiropractic care I had been receiving. I had been a chiropractic patient for over twenty-six years. In my situation, I just made sure I was getting evaluated by my chiropractor at least once per week.

I was finally ready to begin my journey, and I was very excited to get started. All of my preparations, charts, and precautions to ensure my continued well being as I progressed through the program had been completed. It was time to get off my backside and put everything that I had planned into motion.

Walking Away From Obesity

In order for a person to lose a substantial amount of weight and then maintain the accomplishment over a lifetime, it requires a major commitment from the individual to change his or her lifestyle. A weight problem has to be addressed properly and any attempt to manage a condition such as this without making an honest effort to change your lifestyle is probably going to be a waste of your time and quite possibly a hazard to your health.

In this chapter I will explain to readers my walking routine and the benefits that were yielded from this campaign. Through a regular program of walking, I was able to accomplish my weight loss goal of losing seventy pounds in seven months.

To begin with, I made my walking routine one of the most important items in my life. Walking became just as important as my career. I made a decision right from the beginning that I would never skip a day once I started the program. At its peak, my walking routine consisted of a sixty minute workout that covered a distance of approximately three and a half miles. I would perform this walk two times per day on Sunday, Tuesday, Thursday, and Saturday, and one time per day on Monday, Wednesday, and Friday. I would walk seven days a week.

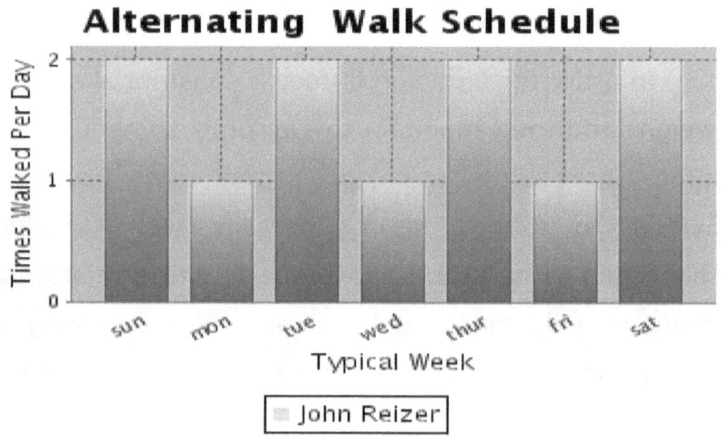

I began my program on January 10, 2007. During the first month, I was unable to walk the peak distance so I began with a half mile in the morning and then a half mile in the evening. After the first month, I was able to gradually increase the distance I walked to one mile per session. By the beginning of March, I had reached my peak distance of three and a half miles per session. From the beginning of March, 2007 – August

31, 2007, I walked approximately 10.5 miles every two days for a total distance of 157 miles per month.

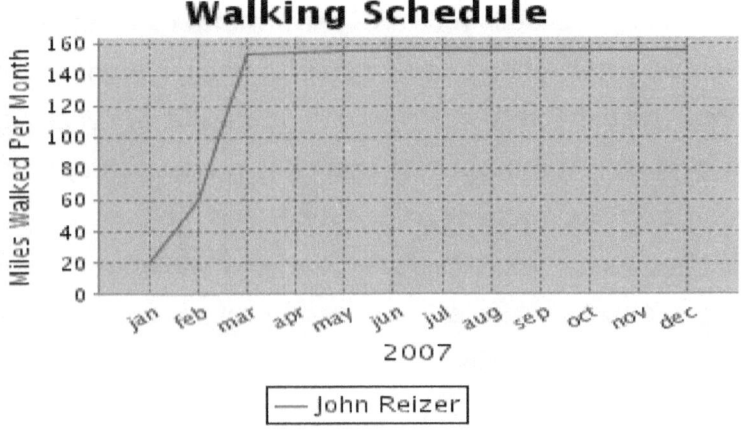

Walking Schedule

As I mentioned previously, I broke up my walking routine into three and a half mile sessions. The first session took place in the morning. On the days that I walked twice in the same day, the second session usually took place later in the evening.

The reason I walked two times per day was to keep my metabolism constantly elevated so that I could burn kilocalories more efficiently. I would schedule my walks approximately twelve hours a part in order to accomplish this strategy. My rationale for walking only one session on day one and then two sessions on day two was to try and confuse the body so that it would have a more difficult time adjusting its metabolic rate to a lower kilocalorie burning level.

The human body is a highly intelligent and adaptive organism. It will attempt to do whatever it deems necessary to survive a particular situation. If your body senses you are performing exercise on a regular basis, and it determines that your workouts fit into a predictable pattern, it will figure out a clever way to minimize the output of energy it requires supporting your exercise routines. Because I was able to change the frequency and the distance of my walking program very often, I was able to produce a much more efficient metabolism on a daily basis.

The Many Benefits of Walking

There are so many benefits associated with walking. In my opinion it is the most logical exercise program to embrace because it is a form of activity that almost anyone can perform. Walking programs can vary in their intensities and I want my readers to understand that at no time whatsoever did I feel like I walked at a pace that was super intense. My walking pace was brisk and it made me feel like I was getting a great workout.

The human being was made to walk. Without a doubt, walking is the most natural form of exercise a person can perform. Walking long distances creates minimal adverse effects on the joints of the body and the stress that it produces on other physiological systems is negligible.

Walking also improves the body's circulation which allows increased levels of oxygenated blood to get to organs, tissues, and cells. People who have sufficient circulation enjoy healthier lives. An organ or system that is not receiving adequate levels of blood, due to circulatory challenges, may suffer permanent damage which can lead to partial or total organ failure.

One of the best benefits of walking is that this form of exercise helps to create lean muscles throughout your entire body. Lean muscles will help boost your metabolism to an extremely high level which will ultimately help you burn calories and fat faster.

Walking also energizes your body. It makes you feel alive and refreshed. The increased oxygen that it provides to your entire body causes many people to feel as if they have a lot more energy.

Recent studies have indicated that walking will help your body to fight off certain diseases. It is now believed by many healthcare experts that the immune system functions better in people who regularly exercise or take part in activities such as a walking program.

Another great benefit of walking is that it helps people handle stress more effectively. Stress is always present in our lives. It is impossible to reduce or eliminate stress in a person's life altogether. What is possible however, is finding clever ways to improve the way that the body adapts to the various forms of stress it encounters. Walking and other forms of exercise can help people to better adapt to the various stresses they regularly deal with.

Prolonged walking campaigns strengthen and improve cardiovascular performance over a person's lifetime. If you want to greatly reduce your chances of having to deal with heart problems later in your life, you should maintain a regular healthy walking program.

One of the best things about walking is that people of all ages can take part in this type of activity. By modifying the pace and the distance of a specific routine, most people can derive some health benefits from a walking program.

Perhaps the most attractive thing I can write about walking is that this type of activity is absolutely free. Walking on a daily basis will not negatively impact a person's budget. Your only expense is possibly purchasing a good pair of sneakers. I also recommend a comfortable outfit that provides warmth in the winter months and is not too hot in the summertime. I usually take with me a bottle of water so that I can keep myself hydrated and I also like to carry a "walking stick" to deter any wild life or neighborhood pets that might cross my path.

My Walking Course & Routine

The daily course that I walked was in my immediate neighborhood and it provided me with an assortment of hills to conquer. This subdivision was rather large and it had long and winding roads with heavily wooded properties. It was ideal for what I wanted to be able to accomplish. The only additional equipment I carried on my person, on certain occasions, was a small flashlight so I could see what was on the road in the early mornings when it was still dark.

As soon as I began to walk, I immediately felt as if I had increased levels of energy. In general, I just felt great and I always looked forward to getting outside and on the course so that I could collect my thoughts and preview or review the day that was in front of me or the one that had just passed.

Before I would begin each of my walking sessions, I would do a few stretching exercises just to wake up my muscles. The actual walk was divided into three stages. During the first stage, *(the warm up)* I would start off walking slow and I would continue this type of pace for about 200 yards. The second stage *(the main course)* was the meat of my walk and I would try to maintain a nice brisk pace during this part of the routine. The final stage *(the cool down)* was a chance for my body to walk at a slower pace during the last 200

Dr. John Reizer

yards, before I completed the exercise session. I would also do some light stretching after the walk had been completed. *(Please refer to the pre and post exercise images below.)*

Pre and Post Stretching Exercises

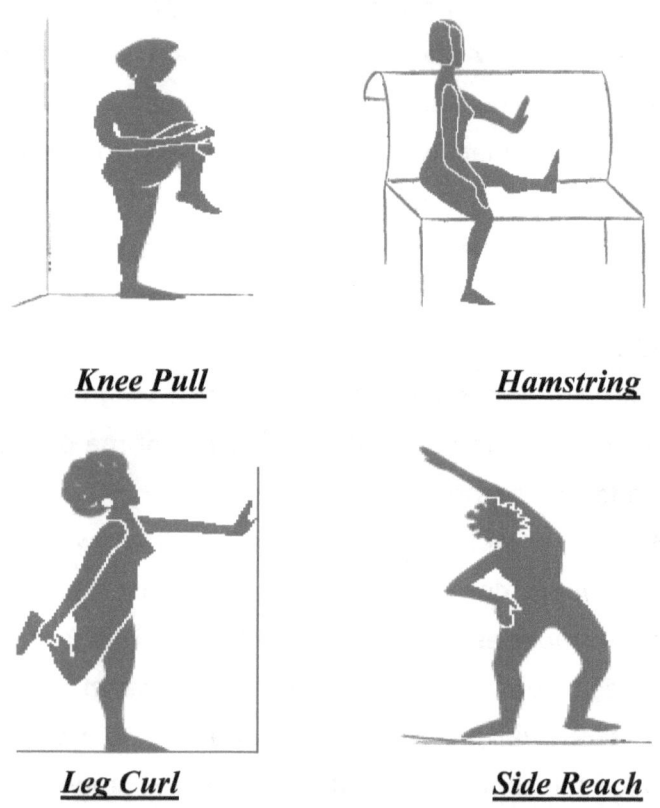

Knee Pull   ***Hamstring***

Leg Curl   ***Side Reach***

It Pays to be Persistent

Those individuals who are persistent in life are usually the most successful people in a given endeavor.

The only difference between a person who is successful at something and a person who is not successful is their attitude and level of determination in approaching their goals. The successful person is able to get off the ground one more time than the person who is not able to succeed. I am a firm believer in the concept that good things will eventually come to those people who do not give up. In my opinion, it is virtually impossible to become a failure at anything if you refuse to throw in the towel. I also believe that the only people who ever fail are those individuals who give up on becoming successful.

You must be completely committed to your walking routine. You cannot let anything in your life distract you from your program. It has to be that important to you and you will definitely have to rearrange certain priorities in your life to stay on track. There will be times when you wake up, early in the morning, and you will not feel like walking. There will be those moments after a long and tiring work day when you will contemplate whether you should skip an exercise session. Do your program as originally planned, without any interruptions. Make your walking program one of the most important items on your daily "to do" list. By regularly performing your exercise sessions, you will automatically create positive habits that are very difficult to stop. Once these habits are in place, you will be totally committed to your routine.

Eating my way back to 175 Pounds

The strategy that I used for the nutritional part of my *waist away* program was based on six common sense components that I believed were extremely important. The first component was a total adherence to my new policy of adding as many healthy foods to my daily diet as possible. While this process was taking place, I had to simultaneously remove all of the unhealthy products I had been previously consuming. The second component of my plan was a drastic increase in my veggies and fruits. The third component called for the removal of as many processed foods as possible, including the elimination of all diet products and artificial sweeteners. The fourth component of the plan was to decrease my portion sizes at each meal. Component number five required me to eat a different number of kilocalories each day, and the final component of my nutritional plan required me to eat a wider variety of healthy foods.

I had been eating unhealthy foods for so long that I had to reeducate my body and brain so that I could recognize what was actually healthy and what was not.

One of the biggest challenges I had to face was my own distorted perception of what an adequate portion size was. My idea of a single portion of a certain type of food was a lot different than what an actual portion or recommended serving looked like.

When I activated my new plan, I learned to become very proficient at measuring quantities of food with a measuring cup, and I also learned how to become an avid reader of nutritional labels. I paid very close attention to the process of measuring out all of my food, and because of this I knew the exact amount of kilocalories I was consuming at each meal.

Prior to my discovery of the measuring cup, I would regularly overeat at just about every meal. For example, I would come home from my private practice or the college where I was working and I would sit down to a large supper that my wife had prepared. She would frequently serve pasta at my request. It was not difficult for me to consume an entire pound of spaghetti or penne macaroni with a heavy sauce at one sitting. After polishing off the main course, I would routinely feast on a couple of slices of chocolate cake with vanilla ice cream. After working on the word processor for a few hours, I would be back in the kitchen snacking on something else. This was a common occurrence and I routinely practiced similar dietary habits at breakfast and lunch.

Adding Healthy Foods to my Diet

I needed to add as many healthy foods as possible to my diet. The first category that I decided to tackle was fruits. I began to eat a healthy selection of fruits every day (at least 5 servings). Whenever possible, I always made an attempt to get the freshest fruits available for that particular season. I always tried to stay away from canned fruits as well as fruit juices.

Increasing my consumption of veggies was also a major part of my strategy. I consumed a lot of spinach, broccoli, kale, romaine lettuce and other dark leafy greens. I also dressed up my salads with carrots, cucumbers, peppers, onions, tomatoes, etc. My total daily vegetable consumption went from zero or trace amounts up to 5 – 6 servings per day.

The next category I worked on was my consumption of various meats (proteins). I made a firm commitment to eat a lot of lean meats and poultry products. I had my wife prepare these foods by grilling them. I wanted to avoid all fried foods in my new diet. On a number of occasions, I would also vary my protein intake with some tuna and salmon dishes. My goal was to consume approximately 5.5 – 7.0 ounces of various meats per day.

My next outlined objective was to regularly consume about 6 – 8 ounces of whole grain breads and or cereals each day. In addition to this, I made sure that I consumed approximately 1 – 2 cups of non-fat milk with my cereals in order to acquire some much needed calcium.

Eliminating Unhealthy Foods

I had been consuming very large portions of desserts, as well as other food products that contained added sugars. Many of the fats that I had been regularly including in my diet were originating from unhealthy sources such as hydrogenated oils and margarine. I had also developed a large appetite for Mexican food which was very high in fat content.

Through the last 7-8 years, I had definitely become a big consumer of potato chips and other non healthy snacks. A bag of chips at lunch, a couple of candy bars during the afternoon, some packages of crackers before sitting down to have supper, and before I was done with the day I had really packed on some low quality kilocalories. I had to work really hard to stop this type of abuse that I was putting my body through. It was amazing that I had not put on even more weight than I had.

Fortunately, about seven years earlier I had done something that was very good for my health. I had stopped drinking all soft drinks. Included in my resolution not to drink soda was an additional commitment I had made to permanently avoid any diet products which contained various artificial sweeteners. I had done some research on these products and had come to the conclusion (my own opinion of course) that they were not good for me. I believed that these artificial sweeteners actually caused me to crave certain types of unhealthy foods. I had no concrete, scientific proof to back up my feelings about artificial sweeteners, but I knew what my cravings felt like during the span of time that I had consumed these products. If I had not given up soft drinks years earlier, I would have been 25-35 pounds heavier than I was in January, 2007.

My Daily Caloric Intake Profile

The actual amount of calories that I decided to consume on a daily basis was determined from running a mathematical calculation which was based on my body size and weight in January, 2007. I also took into consideration the new level of physical activity I was planning to perform.

According to the United States Department of Agriculture, I needed to consume between 3,000 – 3,200 kilocalories per day to maintain my January, 2007 weight of 245 pounds. This calculation, which I obtained from an interactive program on www.mypyramid.gov, took into account my inactive and sedentary lifestyle. I had already been eating, on a regular basis, this amount of kilocalories. The result of the calculation demonstrated to me that even at the very low level of activity I had been performing during that time period, my body was still burning 3,200 kilocalories each day. If you read the chapter where I discussed metabolism, you will remember that I wrote about how the body continues to burn kilocalories even when a person is sleeping or watching television. Because I was eating approximately 3,200 kilocalories each day and my body was burning the same amount of fuel, I continued to maintain my weight, at that time, which was 245 pounds.

I wanted to consume the number of kilocalories per day that would maintain the weight of a 175 pound male who was 5'11 inches tall. I plugged in the data and calculated the results which revealed that in order for me to maintain a weight of 175 pounds I would need to consume 2,800 kilocalories every day. This amount was reflective of a male at my age that was performing between 30 – 60 minutes of exercise per day.

I decided to lower my caloric intake value to 1,750 – 2,000 kilocalories per day. I felt that this amount of kilocalories would sustain my body in a healthy manner and I could always adjust the caloric intake accordingly if I felt that my food supply was becoming inadequate.

In January of 2007, with my new level of physical activity taken into careful consideration, I knew my body would theoretically burn 22,400 kilocalories each week. I also knew that I would be consuming 12,950 kilocalories in a week's time which would leave me with a 9,450 kilocalorie deficit at the end of every week. This translated into a potential weight loss of approximately 2.7 pounds per week if you rationalize that it takes 3,500 kilocalories in one direction or the other to add or lose one pound.

Consuming a Different Number of Calories Each Day

Another strategy I regularly employed was to flip flop the number of kilocalories I would consume on a daily basis. On one day I would eat 2,000 kilocalories and on the next day I would only consume 1,750 kilocalories. This would average out to a 1,875 kilocalorie diet per day. I did this in an effort to prevent my body's metabolism from discovering a specific pattern of decreased caloric intake that would be generated from my *waist away* program. I ultimately wanted my metabolism to continue to burn its fuel at the highest level possible.

The final strategy I wrote into my program was to create a *cheat day* that could be thrown into my caloric intake profile. I utilized a *cheat day* to reward myself for sticking to my *waist away* program and also to help throw the body's metabolism off track. On my *cheat day* I would still eat ultra healthy foods, but I would intentionally eat a much higher number of good quality kilocalories than I would on any other day of that particular month. My rationale was simply that I felt the body's metabolism would raise its calorie burning rate as a result of the higher intake of kilocalories. As long as I followed my blueprint and stuck to my regular caloric intake profile for the remainder of the days in the month, I knew I would see positive results in regards to attaining my body's overall weight loss objectives.

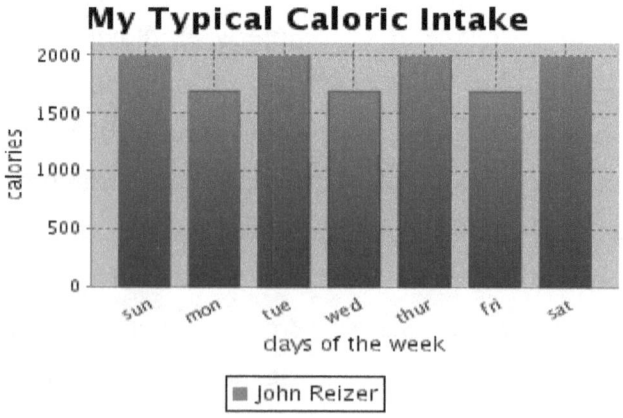

I believe that the strategies I used in the *waist away* program were successful in helping me keep my metabolism running at a higher rate than it normally would. The manner in which I consumed kilocalories, along with the other strategies I used in my walking program, allowed me an opportunity to achieve a sustained period of weight loss without harmful side effects. I also believe that as a result of the strategies I employed, I was able to see a more accelerated weight loss pattern with fewer plateaus (periods of not losing weight) being observed as I charted my progress over time.

Charting My Progress over Time

One of the best ways to determine if your goals are going to be met is to measure the level of progress you are making in regards to the objective in question at various intervals of time.

I was very aware that all of the preparations, strategies and hard work I had placed in this project would be completely meaningless unless I was able to stay committed to my cause and make this program work for me and my family.

I decided back in January, 2007 to keep a weekly journal of my progress. I wanted to document and record each pound that I planned to lose. If I could make my *waist away* program work for me, I would ultimately save my life. I had no choice but to succeed and that is exactly what I planned to do!

In the months of January – August, 2007 I underwent a fantastic physical transformation. As each day passed, I became more in tune with my body and as the days became weeks and the weeks became months, I gradually, over time, began to shed the weight that had held me captive for over 8 years.

In the beginning of January, 2007 I weighed 245 pounds and by the end of August, 2007 I weighed 175 pounds. As I indicated before, when I started my program, I kept a weekly journal of my progress. I was able to keep very accurate records and I have included these journal entries in this portion of the book.

January 10 – 17, 2007:

Whenever I begin a new venture, I usually do so with a lot of enthusiasm. This project was not an exception as I embraced my new lifestyle with a lot of energy and enthusiasm. This week created a lot of sore muscles and the realization that my idea of a portion size is very much out of line with reality. This is going to be a hell of a lot more difficult than I had originally anticipated. My total weight loss for the first week was 2 pounds. My weight as of January 17 is 243 pounds.

January 18 – 24, 2007:

This was another tough week for me. I really dislike getting up so early in the morning. I feel exhausted most of the time and the weather has been pretty cold. I have developed some blisters on my feet, and I feel like I am dying from starvation. I am eating healthy foods everyday. I am constantly rotating my intake of food each day between 1,750 and 2,000 kilocalories. I am also trying to drink as much bottled water as possible. I know that this is good for flushing out the toxins that can build up in the body. I lost 2 more pounds this week and I currently weigh 241 pounds as of this entry.

January 25 – 31, 2007:

My legs and arms feel a little better as I am walking. I think that I am beginning to feel a bit stronger during my walking routine. I actually feel a lot more energized after my walks and I am not as hungry during the day. I have been eating Raisin Bran cereal and a lot of fresh fruit for breakfast, and it really tastes pretty good. I am encouraged because I lost another 2 pounds and I now weigh 239 pounds.

February 1 – 7, 2007:

I am definitely getting into this routine. I have felt very good all week and I am actually looking forward to walking each day. My weight fluctuated a little this week but by the end of the week I had trimmed off another 2 pounds. I am down to 237 pounds.

February 8 – 14, 2007:

My wife's grandmother died this week and I had to make a trip down to Margate, Florida with the family. I managed to get in some exercise but was not able to walk my normal course each day. We also made a stop at Disney World on the way back to South Carolina for my daughter. This was actually a good thing because I walked all over the "Magic Kingdom" getting in a lot of quality miles. I was also very careful what I consumed in the way of food. I have become very strict with myself lately and I believe that I am starting to build healthy habits that reinforce my program. I lost a total of two more pounds this week. My weight is now at 235 pounds and I have lost a total of 10 pounds since I began my journey on January 10.

February 15 – 21, 2007:

I'm making progress, feeling stronger and more energized than before. My daughter and wife have colds and I just hope that I do not come down with what they have because I don't want to screw up my routine. I lost 1 pound this week and I am now at a weight of 234 pounds.

February 22 – 28, 2007:

February is over and I lost 2 more pounds this week. I lost a total of 7 pounds during the month of February. I currently weigh 232 pounds. It is beginning to get warm in South Carolina and the grass is already growing. I'll be mowing the lawn soon. I am actually trying to get in touch with the company that cut my lawn last year. I will hire them to cut the lawn and I will concentrate on my walking program.

March 1 – 7, 2007:

I think that I have hit a little plateau this week. I lost 2 pounds on the first day of the month and then I actually gained a pound. By the end of the week I lost the weight again. I am a little frustrated, but hanging in there. I am committed to this plan and nothing is going to stop me from accomplishing my objective. My weight is now 230 pounds.

March 8 – 14, 2007:

This was another good week. I am continuously dropping my weight. I finished the week with a weight of 228 pounds. I am noticing a difference in the way my clothes are fitting. They're beginning to feel looser. I can see that there is a slight difference in the way my face looks. I am definitely looking thinner in my face.

March 15 – 21, 2007:

I am disappointed because I did not lose any weight this week. I have been weighing myself just about every day and I am watching my weight go up and down. I feel like a damn yoyo on a string. I know that I have hit a plateau once again. I continue to follow my game plan and I've been mixing up my foods as well as my caloric intake every other day. I just have to remain patient and realize that losing weight takes time. I have to remember that I didn't get this way overnight and I am not going to get out of this situation overnight either. I am still at a weight of 228 pounds on March 21, 2007

March 22 – 28, 2007:

I have been walking approximately 155 miles each week and I know that I am doing my body a tremendous service. I dropped 3 more pounds this week and I feel as if my metabolism is definitely responding to my walking schedule as well as my strategy of alternating the calories I consume. My weight is now 225 pounds and I have lost a total of 20 pounds since January 10, 2007.

March 29 – April 4, 2007:

The warm weather is back. I had a very productive week and I am very focused on my goals. I lost a total of 3 pounds in one week and I continue to feast on veggies and fruits like never before. I believe that this is about the healthiest I have ever been as far as consuming nutritious foods. I love salads and I have been eating them often along with personal, small pizzas. My wife makes the pizzas and they're only about 400 kilocalories. I usually have two of these pizzas for dinner with a large salad. I now weigh 222 pounds.

April 5 – 11, 2007:

I hit another plateau this week and I have not lost any weight. The good news is that I didn't gain any weight back. My exercise program is doing well and the diet I am on is great. I am not walking around hungry at all. I could maintain this type of a regiment indefinitely. I feel great! My weight is 222 pounds.

April 12 – 18, 2007:

The pace of my walk has become very brisk and I feel as if I am beginning to get in very good shape. I know that I have a lot of weight to lose but I feel as if my level of progress is accelerating each week. I lost 3 more pounds and I am down to a weight of 219 pounds.

April 19 – 25, 2007:

I'm doing very well this week. I lost 2 additional pounds over the past 7 days and I am feeling pretty light on my feet. People at work, as well as some of my patients, have asked me if I am losing weight. I tell them that, "I can't find it anywhere." I now weigh 217 pounds.

April 26 – May 2, 2007:

I just celebrated my 15 wedding anniversary with my wife. I also dropped another 3 pounds this past week and that makes me extremely happy. We celebrated our anniversary and went out to a nice restaurant. I behaved at the restaurant and stuck to my plan. I continue to eat ultra healthy foods and I can see the results in the way I look and feel. I currently weigh 214 pounds.

May 3 – 10, 2007:

It has been warm recently and I think the summer weather is almost here. I am feeling very strong and my wife has informed me that my sleep apnea has stopped. She tells me that I am sleeping sound and there has not been any snoring. I am thankful for this. I lost no weight this week but that's part of the process I am going through. I currently weigh 214 pounds.

May 11 – 17, 2007:

I have had another great week with my program. I lost 2 more pounds and everything is going according to plan. I have lost a significant amount of weight already but I am still not even at the half way point. My waist size for pants is now a 38 and I currently weigh 212 pounds.

May 18 – 24, 2007:

My daughter just graduated from Kindergarten and we are officially on summer vacation at my house. I like this time of the year and for the first time, in a while, I feel like I have some energy to enjoy the outdoors. I lost 2 more pounds and my weight is gradually inching downward. I currently weigh 210 pounds.

May 25 – 31, 2007:

I just got back from Myrtle Beach, South Carolina where we had a few days of rest and relaxation. We rented a beautiful ocean front condominium and had a lot of fun in the sun. I walked on the beach and up and down the streets that ran parallel to the coastline. I followed and maintained my diet plan during this short trip. I did utilize one cheat day on Saturday the 28 of May. I must have dumped a lot of water weight because I dropped almost 6 pounds since last week. I think all of the running around on the beach, with my daughter, helped facilitate the extra weight loss that has occurred. I don't really want to drop weight that fast but I do feel very healthy and energized. I currently weigh 204 pounds.

June 1 – 7, 2007:

This has been an exceptionally good week. My energy levels are increasing each day and I am really shedding the pounds pretty fast at this point. I lost 4 additional pounds since my last journal entry and I currently weigh 200 pounds. I am ready to cross the magical 200 pound mark. Bring it on!

June 8 – 14, 2007:

I just finished the spring quarter at the college where I teach. I am now on summer vacation for the next month and it feels great to have a break to look forward to. I feel pretty good as I am now below 200 pounds. I lost 2 pounds this week and my exercise routine is going well. I currently weigh 198 pounds. I have lost a total of 47 pounds since January 10.

June 15 – 21, 2007:

My wife and I have been walking together since my vacation from the college started. She is in very good shape and enjoys the routine I have put together. She also has a super healthy diet and this helps me to focus and stay on track. I am every bit as committed to my program today as I was back in January. I lost 2 pounds this week and currently weigh 196 pounds.

June 22 – 28, 2007:

Tomorrow we are going to celebrate my wife's 37th birthday. I continue to take off the excess weight that I have accumulated over the past 7 years. This week I took my daughter Kayla to the movies and we had a great time. We are all getting excited because next week we are going back to Myrtle Beach to celebrate the 4th of July holiday. My workouts and diet are really making me waist away (pardon the play on words). This sounds like a good title for a new book. Maybe I'll sit down and write a book featuring my waist away program when I finally reach my target weight of 175 pounds. I lost 3 pounds this week and I now weigh 193 pounds.

June 29 – July 5, 2007:

I'm on vacation in Myrtle Beach and the weather has been just perfect. The ocean front condo is wonderful and we have been dining at some good restaurants. I have maintained my diet plan as well as my walking routine and I feel extremely confident as I walk into various restaurants and look over a menu. I feel that I can easily pick something, from any menu, that is healthy and good for me no matter where I happen to be. I lost 1 pound this week and currently weigh 192 pounds.

July 6 – 12, 2007:

I am slowly but surely closing in on my target. I have lost 3 pounds this week and I weigh 189 pounds. I started teaching at school once again as the summer vacation has ended. Many of the faculty members and students are amazed at the amount of weight I have lost. They seem to believe that I have lost this weight in the last month. I have assured them that this has been a gradual process and that I am perfectly healthy.

July 13 – 19, 2007:

My Waist Away Program is so much a part of my lifestyle at this point in time that it is hard for me to refer to it as a program. I have changed the way that I live and I believe that I am much healthier than ever before. I have lost 3 additional pounds over the last week. I currently weigh 186 pounds.

July 20 – 26, 2007:

I made some more progress this week as I burned another 3 pounds. The weather has been extremely hot and I find myself walking very early in the mornings and very late at night in an effort to try and stay out of the intense summer heat. I currently weigh 183 pounds.

July 27 – August 2, 2007:

I lost 2 more pounds this week and I am really feeling strong and committed to this process. I can see the finish line in the distance. I am ready to sip some champagne. I currently weigh 181 pounds. My pants (size 36) are fitting very loose at this point. I think I am going to end up in a size 34. This is actually pretty amazing. My brother told me he cannot believe the transformation I have gone through and he is encouraging me to author a new book on my accomplishment.

August 3 – 9, 2007:

The last few pounds are always the most difficult. I am stuck at 181 pounds for the moment but I realize it is only a matter of time before my success is realized. This is an incredible program because I have methodically lost all of this weight, and I did it by just setting my caloric intake to a level that would maintain the weight of a 44 year old man at approximately 175 pounds.

August 10 – 16, 2007:

I am getting anxious as the final couple of pounds are finally coming off. I think my body is acclimating to my new weight and I believe that the journey is almost over. I did lose 3 pounds this week and I now weigh 178 pounds.

August 17 – 23, 2007:

I continue to struggle with the last couple of pounds. My daughter started first grade this week and I am still stuck on 178 pounds. I am making some preparations to write a new book about my weight loss program. I think I will call the book, "Waist Away: How I Lost 70 Pounds in 7 Months without Dangerous Drugs or Surgery." I think that title is catchy. I ran the title by my brother and he liked it as well. I told my wife I wanted to write a new book and she did not look too happy initially, but I think she is coming around and I know in the end she will be supportive of whatever I try to accomplish. When I write a book, I often devote a lot of time to the word processor and she doesn't get to see me as much as she would like to. I told her that I would definitely pace myself and that she should not worry as I would work on the manuscript in the evenings when my daughter and she were sleeping.

August 24 – 31, 2007:

I finally hit my target weight of 175 pounds and I am so happy that I was able to stay focused and reach my ultimate objective. I know that I have saved my life and I feel relieved that I was able to finally hit the 175 mark. Now my mindset shifts to maintaining the weight that I have lost. It gives me a great sense of personal satisfaction to know that I had the ability to stick with my program and I was ultimately successful in accomplishing my weight loss goals.

I was able to create the graphs on the next few pages from the collection of notes that I kept as I charted my weight loss progress over time. These graphs are a relatively accurate depiction of how many pounds I lost during the months that I participated in my *waist away* program.

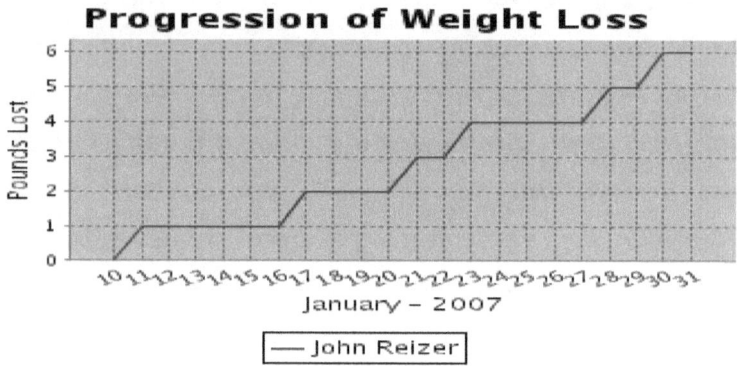

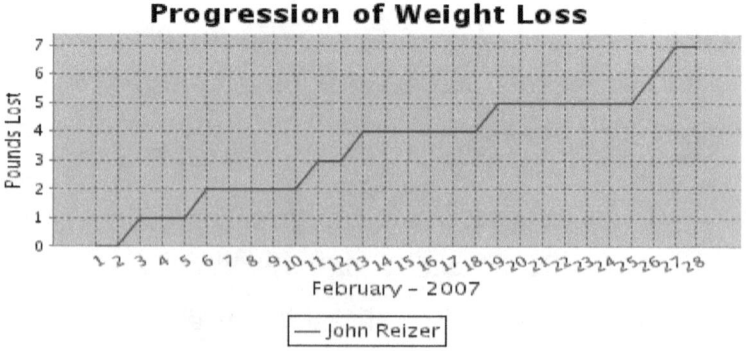

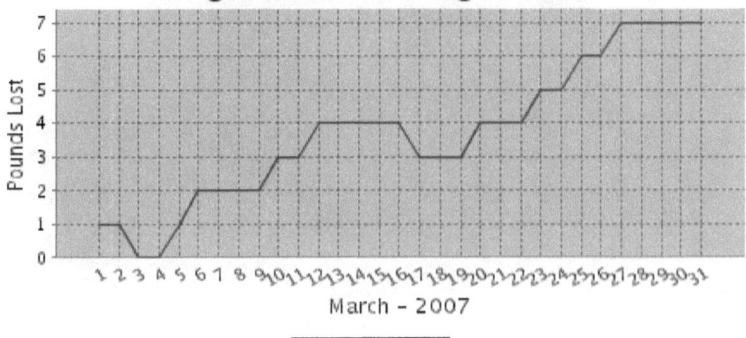

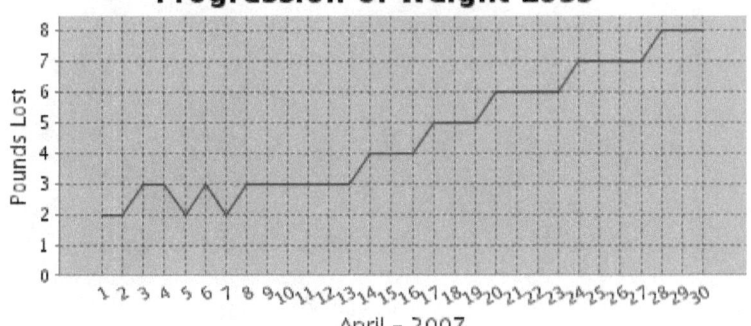

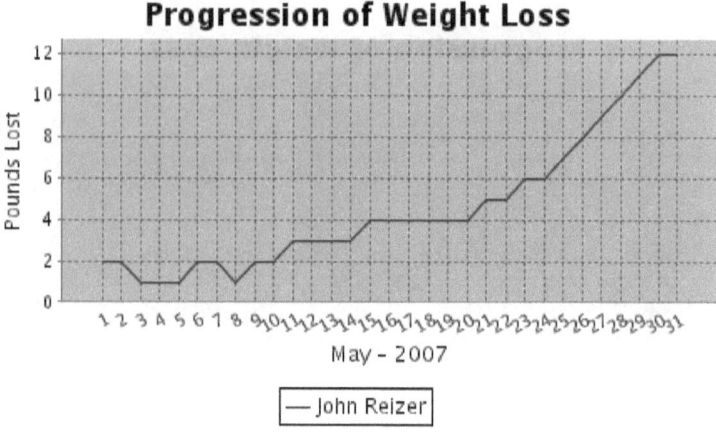

Progression of Weight Loss

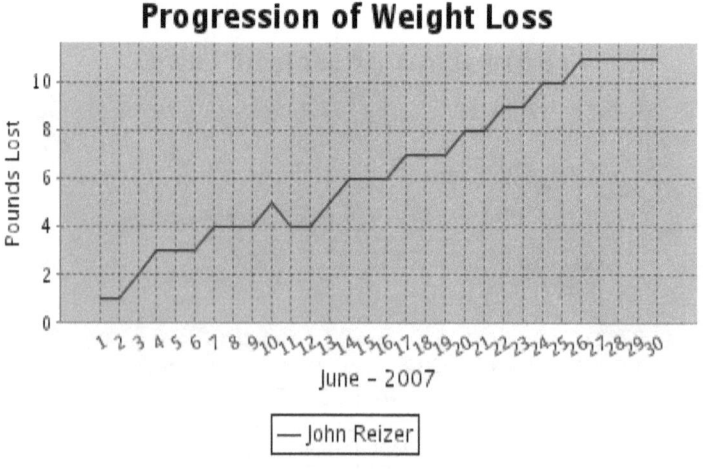

Progression of Weight Loss

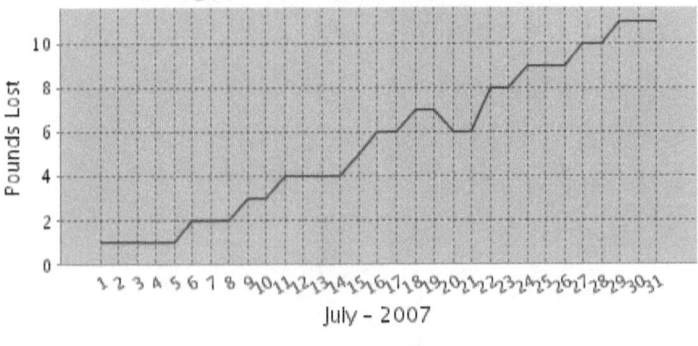

July – 2007

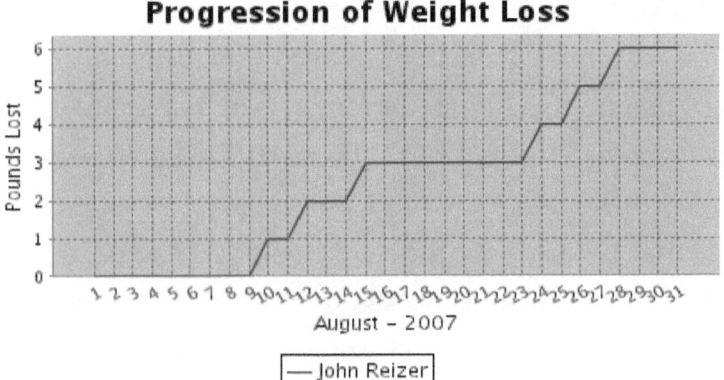

August – 2007

Pictures Don't Lie!

The pictures included in this section of the book were taken by friends and family members. These photographs represent a collection of *"before and after"* images of your author at various social and professional gatherings. Some of the *"after"* photographs were taken by my wife in our home in South Carolina.

In one of these photographs I am wearing size 40 dress pants that were extremely snug on me in the beginning of January, 2007. In reality, I had a hard time getting these pants on and I was actually afraid if I bent over that I would tear a hole in them. In August, 2007 I was able to step into the same pants and I had a lot of material left over. By the end of August, 2007 I was comfortably wearing size 34 pants and I was 70 pounds lighter.

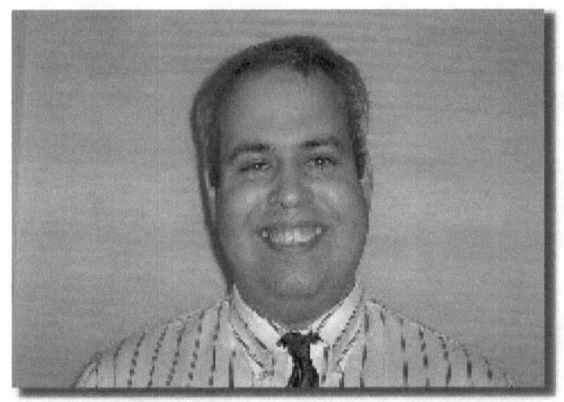

The Author – December, 2002

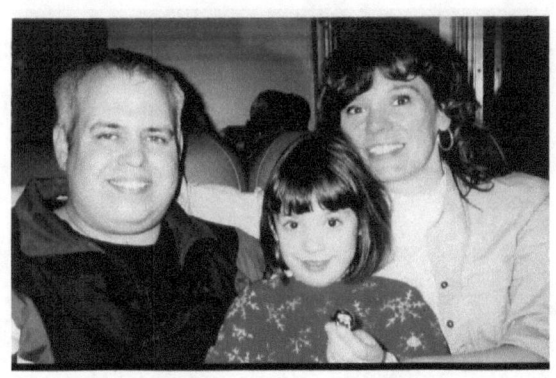

John & Family, December, 2006

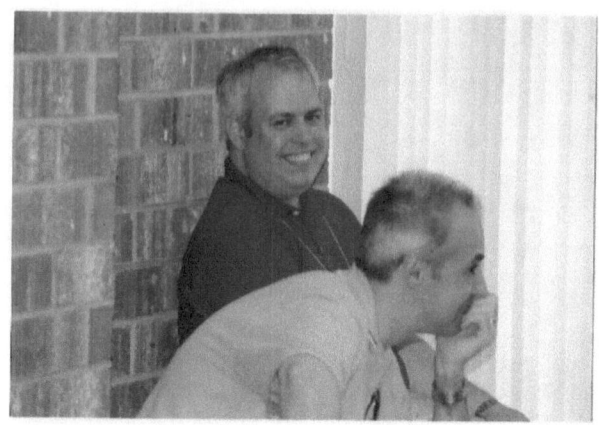

John & Brother Steve – May, 2006

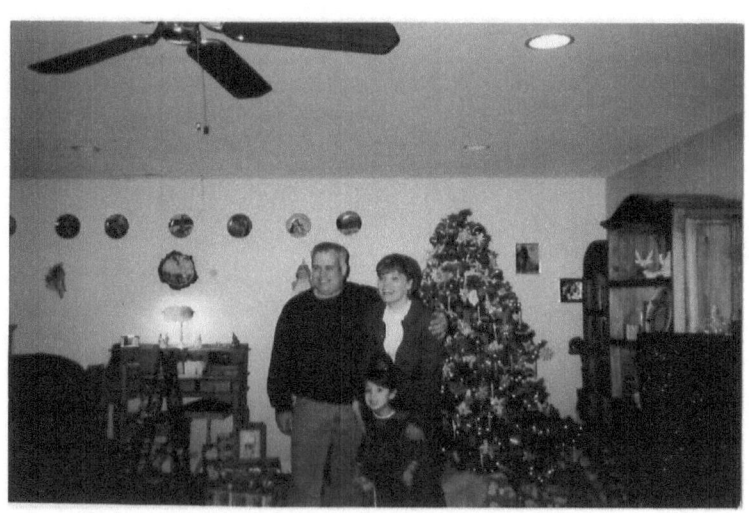

John & Family – December, 2006

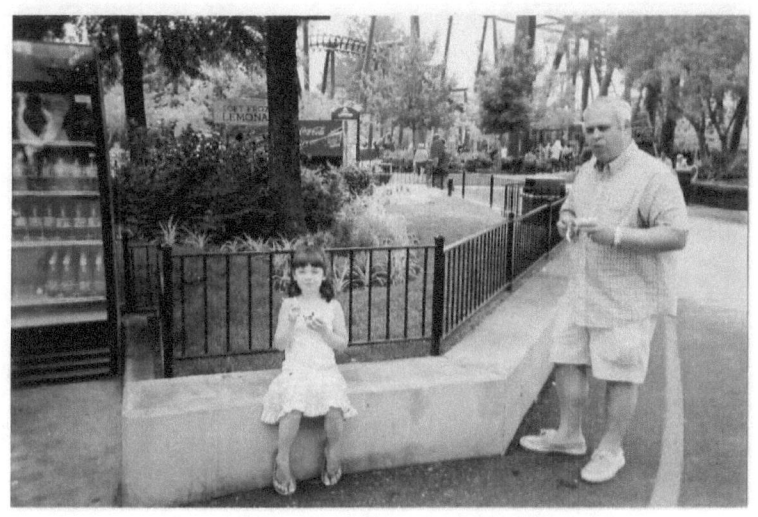

John & Kayla – July, 2006
(Size 40 Pants / Shorts)

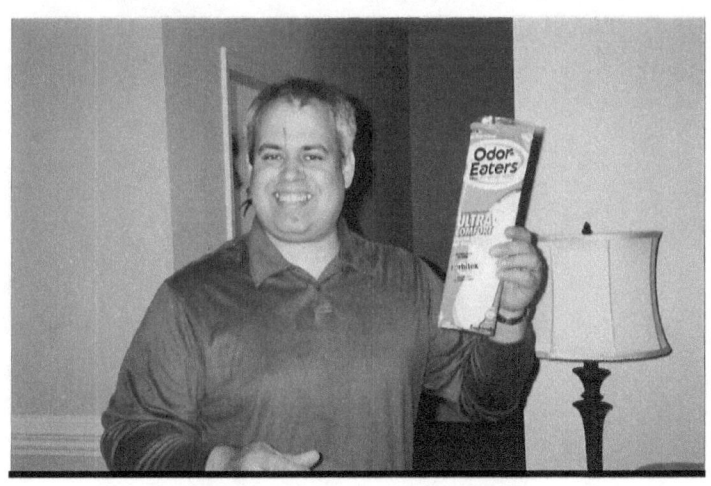

John – December, 2006

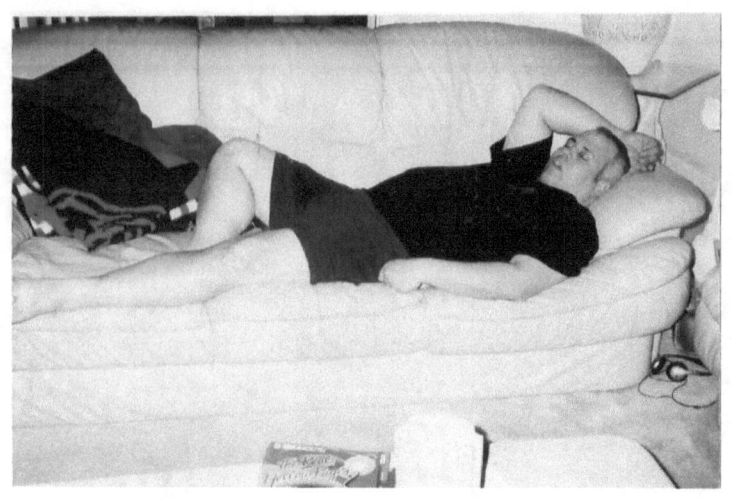

John Sleeping on couch – November, 2006

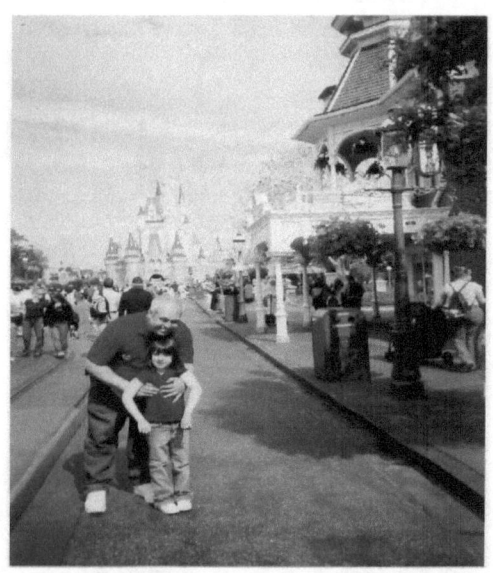

John & Kayla – February, 2007
Disney World – Florida

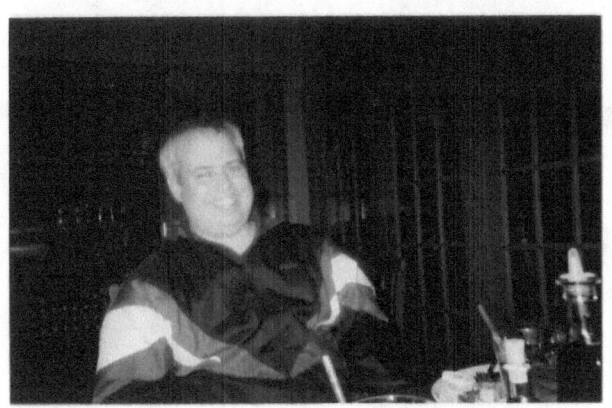

John – September, 2006

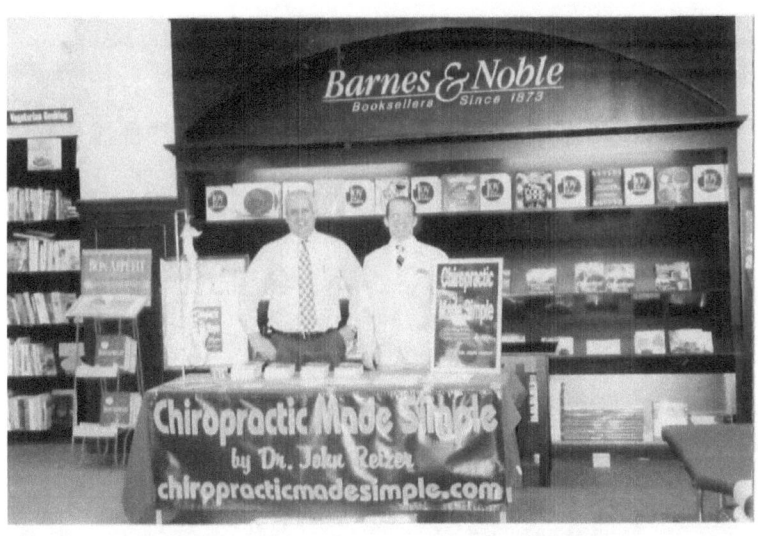

John at Book Signing – January, 2007
(Size 40 Dress Pants)

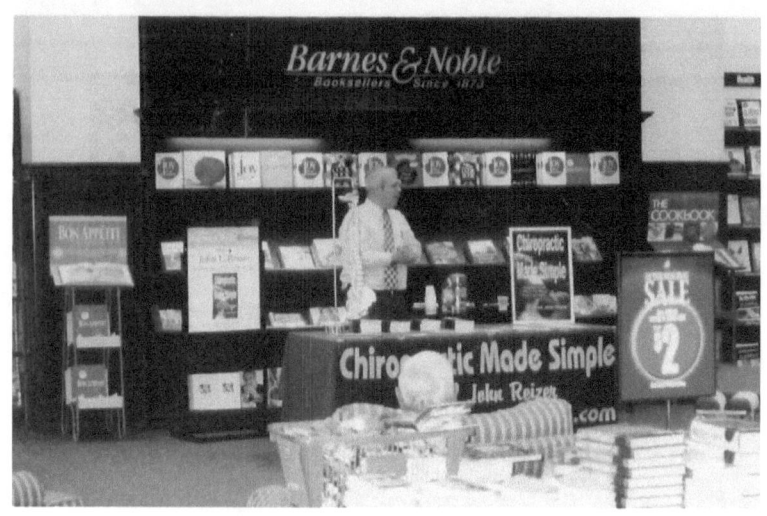

John at Book Signing – January, 2007

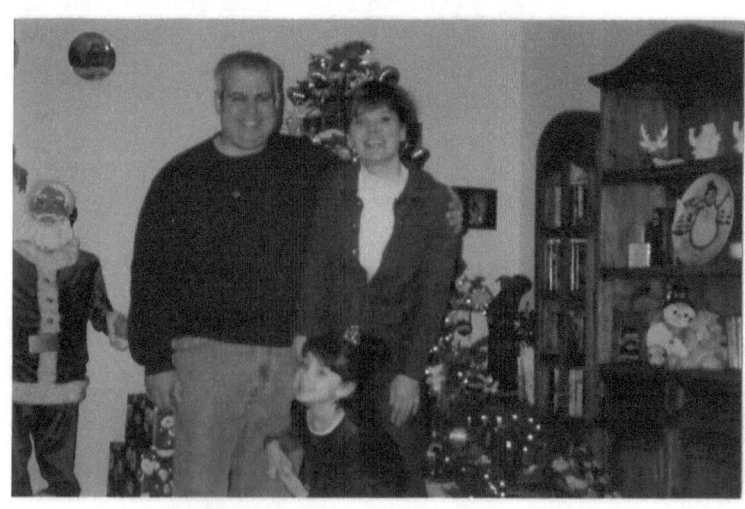

John with Wife Melissa & Kayla – December, 2006
(Size 40 Blue Jeans)

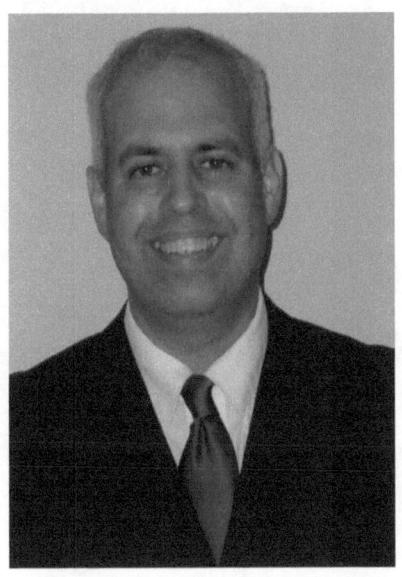

John 70 Pounds lighter – August, 2007

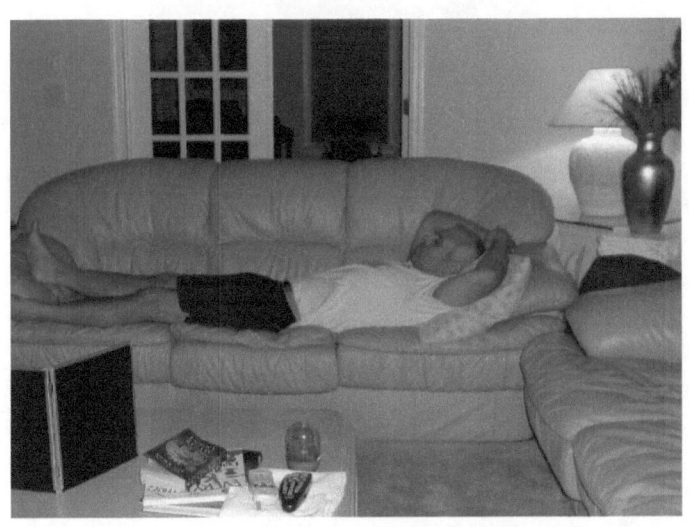

John sleeping on the couch – August, 2007

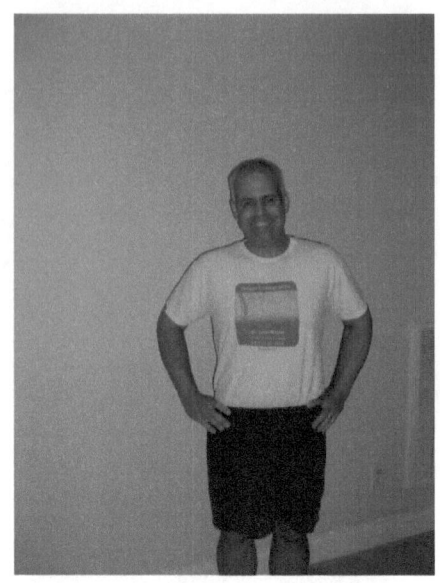

John – August, 2007

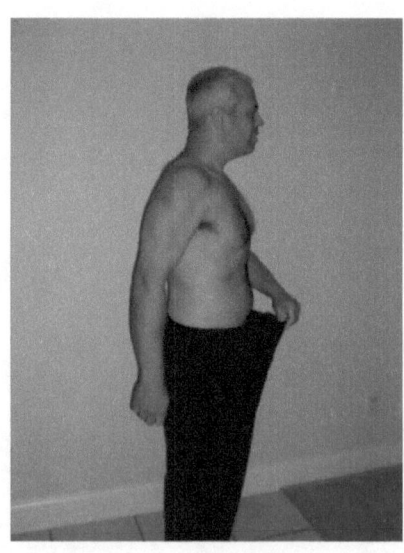

My size 40 pants fit very snug in February, 2007

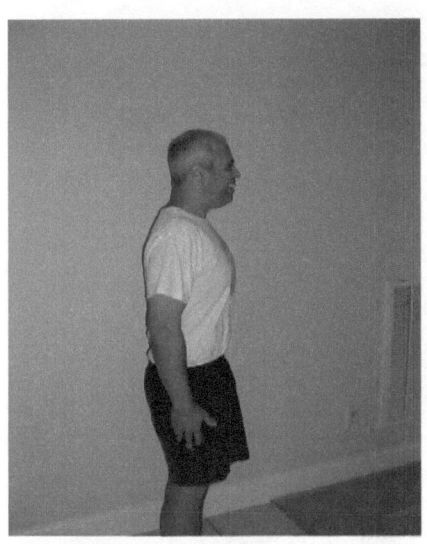

John – 175 pounds & Skinny in August, 2007

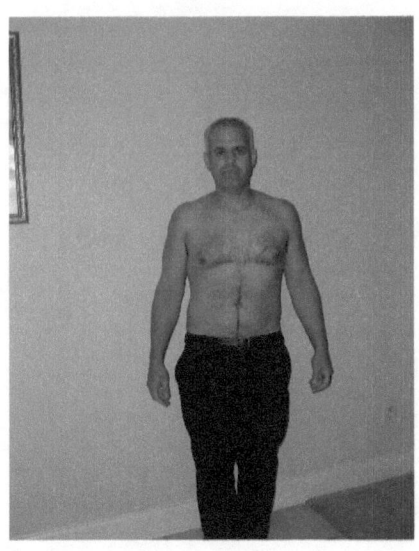

Size 34 Dress Pants in August, 2007

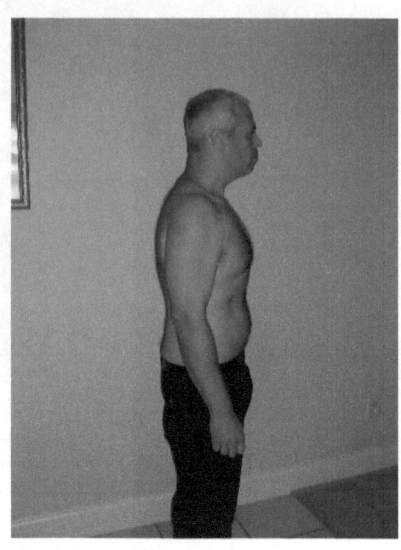

Size 34 Dress Pants in August, 2007

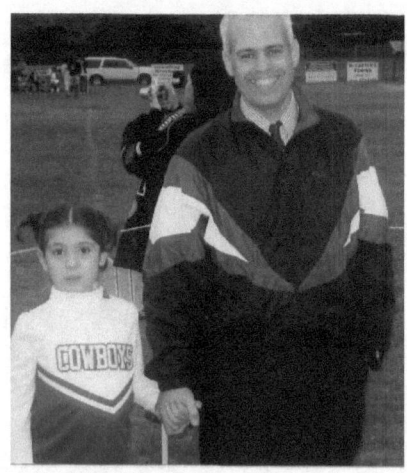

September, 2007

Understanding the Purpose of Food and Changing My Perception of Reality

In retrospect, I can honestly admit to my readers that my eating habits had been absolutely atrocious during the past few years of my life. I could easily compare my mindset, during those years, to that of a train running down a track with no one in the engineer's compartment. The situation had progressed to a point where it was endangering my health and well being. I was completely out of control on many occasions, and I am very thankful for the divine force that was able to tap me on the shoulder and finally wake me up.

My current mindset is 180 degrees opposite from what it once was in the not so distant past. I now look at food with a different set of eyes. I believe that my physical body, as well as my psyche, experienced a beneficial process of transformation.

My attitude not so long ago was that I did not have a weight problem. I could be sitting down, having lunch, and be thinking about what my next meal at dinner was going to feature. I was constantly in deep thought about eating and I was not at all interested in taking part in physical activities.

All of my social events would naturally revolve around food. I realize today that eating is something that is done to nourish the human body and should not be used as a prop within the social arena. While I believe that it is ok to have a healthy meal with friends and family during social gatherings, I also believe that the presence of friends and family members should not be a catalyst for engaging in the consumption of meals when you are not really hungry.

I have re-educated my mind to be more cognizant of the importance and purpose of food for my body. Food is a necessity to sustain and maintain life. It is utilized as a vehicle to nourish the body and it simultaneously maintains the continuity of the physiological processes that ensure our existence. When explained in those terms, it is easy for me to observe in the present how distorted my perception of food was in the past.

America, as a society, has glamorized food and made it the featured event in many social arenas. In the modern era of cable and satellite television programming, it is easy to find various networks that are dedicated to showcasing the preparation and serving of culinary specialties. The food channels are a part of our very own culture. We Americans love to eat food. Just about any event is reason enough to create a feast. If my readers took the time to think about this concept, I think that they would agree that my premise holds true when scrutinized. Think about the different holidays that we celebrate in our country and how food of some sort is always attached to each theme. When I think of the 4th of July, I dream of a hot dog with baked beans and slaw. If I think of Thanksgiving, I have visions of turkey, mashed potatoes and pumpkin pie. Easter Sunday makes me think of ham, and the thought of Christmas makes me think of cookies and pastries. Social events, holidays and large gatherings such as funerals, communions, birthdays, etc., are often associated with food.

Another example of consuming food in conjunction with a social event is going to the movies. People that have just finished a big dinner will routinely purchase tickets to see a movie. Within seconds of entering the theatre, the same people will purchase large containers of popcorn and other snacks. These individuals are not hungry by any stretch of the imagination, but yet they still feel the need to consume the popcorn and snacks because that is what has been programmed into their minds.

Over time, we have been conditioned to respond to certain triggers that have been placed into our domain by multinational corporations. These companies have spent many millions of dollars on advertising campaigns in order to instill this type of psychological trickery into the minds of the various members of our society. It has worked like a charm. When people go to the movies, they expect to pay a lot of money for their snacks and they also expect to eat a lot of popcorn whether they are hungry or not. This is what is expected by most people and because it is expected it has become the perceived reality for the average American consumer.

In order to have success with my *waist away* program, I had to change my own perception of reality and I have to confess that this was not an easy task for me to accomplish. Sometimes however, you gain tremendous strength and determination when you feel like your back is up against a wall and you have nowhere else to go except for one obvious direction that is positioned in front of you. I think that pretty much summed up the way I felt in January, 2007. I had only one direction to head for or I could continue to get heavier and gain so much weight that I would make myself ill.

Perception versus Reality

For many years, I taught a course in chiropractic college called *philosophical applications*. I often discussed with my students the difference between reality and a person's perception of reality. It really is a very fascinating topic and many of the students loved to regularly discuss this material with me. I often told students that what we think is reality is actually our limited perception of reality. I also explained to my students that most citizens, living in a structured society, exist in what I commonly refer to as a "herd mentality." I say this because most people are the disciples of information that they cannot possibly verify. Most members of society rely on so called trusted media sources for all of their information (reality). This information is what literally shapes their opinions about the world they live in. They will take the information from these corporate owned news companies and transfer the data into their own core beliefs. In addition, they will defend these core beliefs with great emotion until the very day they die.

A very interesting company called *Strategic Communications Laboratory* www.scl.cc/home.php, which specializes in helping governments to control the

105

perceptions of citizens in many countries around the world, offers this quote from their official website:

"We live in a world of communication, where perception is very often the reality. Those individuals that control the perceptions are the ones that control virtually everything. Most modern conflicts are based on misaligned perceptions, ideologies, opinions about religion, etc. If a government does not have the tools to manage the perceptions which effect security, defense, finance, tourism, health and foreign relations, then it may well find itself at the mercy of those that do."

Members of our society have been subjected to many types of mind control campaigns. We have to face the uncomfortable fact that many of us watch and are influenced by the very same *media programming* as our neighbors. Many of our own perceptions of the world have been artificially influenced by a constant stream of psychological warfare, directed through a seemingly harmless television (tell – a – vision) set. We do not even get a chance to have our own opinions on most subjects. All major news issues are very neatly spoon fed to a viewer audience, and then carefully summarized by an expert appearing on the telecast. We are subconsciously fed propaganda by corporate controlled news companies. The very same themes are then repeated and supported by television programs and major motion pictures. The themes are also endorsed by professional sports leagues, commercials, talk radio shows, and other media outlets that we plug into.

Learning to Think Outside the Box

As members of society we are regularly encouraged by others not to make waves and to defend the defined borders of what is commonly known as conventional thinking. Those brave souls who venture "outside the box" of conventional thinking, more often than not, will face a heavy dose of criticism from an unforgiving society which never considers leaving the confinement of such a well defined safe zone.

After stepping on my bathroom scale in January, 2007 I immediately knew that I too had become a member of the herd mentality. I was allowing myself to take part in a perception of reality that I had inherently rejected for a substantial portion of my life. Many of the concepts that I regularly lectured about to my students, for so many years had come back to haunt me. I was drowning in a sea of conformity and I did not have the desire to reach out and grab a life vest.

I now understood that the issues which had been adversely affecting me on a personal level had to be dealt with. After a short period of time, I was able to refocus my attention on the items in my life that I could control. I also relearned how to let go of the many obstacles in my life that I could not directly influence.

I was convinced at this point that I had been suffering from a case of job related burnout. It was obviously affecting me personally as well as professionally and ultimately affecting my weight. This was the second time in my life that this condition had grabbed hold of me and caused havoc in my life. I had become so wrapped up in my work at school, and with the various writing projects that consumed so much of my time, I became emotionally and mentally burned out.

It is extremely important for readers to understand that the same attributes which can help an individual become successful in life can also be the key factors in causing the person to become frustrated and filled with emotions of depression and despair. We can all benefit from knowing that our lives are made up of many different parts and that in order for people to be happy and successful they need to create some sort of balance between these parts.

Many people, such as your author, who are goal oriented run into the trap of working themselves into a state of physical and emotional burnout. I am not a psychologist who specializes in this sort of disorder however; I have had an opportunity in my own life to experience, firsthand, the effects of professional burnout on two different occasions.

In order to avoid periods of burnout, which can be very destructive to anyone, you must be able to recognize the various indicators that often accompany this condition. Most of us have probably heard the saying *"The first step in solving a problem is identifying one."* I often wonder if people realize how accurate this statement is. A large number of people who suffer from emotional and physical burnout are not even aware that they have such problems. The condition sneaks up on them while they are busy living their lives. All of a sudden they are in trouble and in need of help. Unfortunately, in many instances help is not available and the people suffering have absolutely nowhere to turn.

Some of the indicators of this condition are discussed in this chapter. If you are able to identify any of these items in your own life, it might be a good idea for you to pay very close attention to the material discussed in this section.

Obviously, symptomatic indicators can vary in their intensities and I am not trying to offer a treatment plan or to provide a specific diagnosis for individuals. This information is to be used for educational purposes only and should not be misinterpreted by the reader as a substitute for a proper psychological evaluation by a qualified professional.

Feelings of Frustration

One of the most common indicators of work related burnout is the presence of frustration within your life. No matter what it is you are trying to accomplish there will be this overwhelming feeling that some powerful force is trying to impede your progress. Feelings of frustration can manifest in your business or work life at the onset of this disorder and then later on will begin to show up in your personal and family life as well.

Daydreaming

Very often, people who are suffering from the effects of burnout will spend a good portion of their time thinking about alternative life or job related scenarios that might be perceived, by such individuals, as being less stressful or perhaps even more exciting than their current life situations. Daydreaming is often utilized by those of us who are suffering from burnout because it provides a temporary form of escapism from various sets of circumstances that have caused problems to take shape in the first place. People who regularly daydream about changes in their lifestyle could quite possibly be suffering from a form of burnout.

Physical and Mental Exhaustion

Another indicator that is often reported by workers plagued with burnout is their constant feelings of being exhausted no matter how much sleep they are able to acquire. In this situation, the persons suffering with these problems will often try to work through the apparent feelings of fatigue only to discover that their physical and mental exhaustion never seems to leave them.

Emotional Meltdowns

Burnout will very often cause individuals to suddenly, and without warning, develop unusual feelings that directly lead to emotional outbursts or fits of rage. These emotional meltdowns are, in many situations, uncontrollable as well as completely unpredictable. The slightest little event could cause sufferers to "snap" into an episode for no apparent reason.

Emotional outbursts can cause many problems in the workplace environment and can eventually feed into the original problem by creating more frustration and an even deeper state of burnout.

Feelings of Depression and Despair

Some of the most intense symptomatic indicators of burnout experienced by persons in the workplace and at home are continuous feelings of depression along with the prevailing attitude that there is little chance for any help within the immediate future. Feelings of this nature can be so strong that some people, experiencing such emotions, often consider drastic actions.

Feelings of Negativity

Strong feelings of negativity will often be present in people who suffer from burnout. Almost everything that these individuals are associated with becomes bathed in an attitude of doom and gloom. People who are usually upbeat and very positive in their daily interactions with family and co-workers are suddenly a cancer within their own environment. The strong negative vibrations these people are harboring are immediately perceived by business associates and family members. The effects of the overall situation are quickly revealed by a number of problems in the home and the workplace which will additionally confirm the presence of a much larger problem over time.

Panic Attacks

Shortness of breath, pain in your chest, a rapid heart beat, indigestion, fatigue and a feeling of impending doom that is lurking over you are just a few of the symptoms associated with having a panic attack. Many people in the world suffer from panic disorders or similar stress related episodes. It would be inaccurate to report that all of these panic disorder cases are directly attributed to a specific category of work related stress. However, it is certainly plausible and a working hypothesis of many psychologists that a substantial number of these cases are a direct result of pressures in the workplace. Keep in mind that many individuals suffering from occupational related burnout are prone to having panic attacks.

Increased Appetite

The cumulative effect of these indicators will often cause an individual to experience an increase in his or her appetite. All of a sudden, the routine of eating more food helps to soothe the pain that is being caused by the large number of problems that we have been discussing. Obviously, increased appetite will eventually lead to excessive weight gain which often reinforces feelings of guilt and causes even more depression. These indicators all seem to feed off one another and become part of a great big vicious cycle that is very difficult to break away from.

It Happened to me in the 90's

I like to think of myself as an optimistic person who is able to pick out the smallest components representing something positive, in an otherwise very bleak situation. I have always positioned my emotional tuner at a setting which was compatible with picking up vibrations that were resonating at higher and more positive frequency ranges.

In the late 90's I experienced a severe case of work related burnout. It was at this time that I became inundated with extreme feelings of negativity that I had not previously experienced. These feelings were obviously triggered by my own obsessive work habits which caused me to experience many of the indicators of burnout that I have been writing about in this chapter. Although this was a very short period of time in my life, it turned out to be a very costly experience from a financial point of view.

As a result of my emotional state of mind during those couple of years, I made decisions to walk away from two very lucrative professional chiropractic practices that I had built from the ground up and to move to an entirely new state in order to begin a career as a college instructor. The negativity which I had experienced during this time of my life, as well as my decision to leave my private practice, was not very representative of my overall personality. These two decisions however, offered me an opportunity to make necessary changes in my life that would eventually allow me the time to rest and recover from the problems I had been suffering from. As it turned out, these decisions would be the most important ones I had ever made. They ultimately gave me an opportunity to balance out those other parts of my life which had been neglected for so many years. The financial loss I experienced, that seemed somewhat traumatic at the time, was a sacrifice I needed to make in order to get my life back on track. A few years later, I was able to recover from my financial woes and suddenly the pain in my wallet magically disappeared. I realize today that the financial concerns that had once been a part of my life were much easier to correct than some of the problems which were affecting my overall health and well being.

Given the same identical set of circumstances, I would have to make the same decisions all over again. It was the only way that I could have successfully eliminated the emotional and physical burnout which I was experiencing at the time.

My most recent experience with job related burnout did not provide me with many of the symptoms that had plagued me years earlier. Nevertheless, I am absolutely convinced that much of my weight gain during the past few years was a direct byproduct of work related burnout.

Preventing Burnout

There are a number of proactive steps that you can take to prevent these problems. Again, it is important to remember that recognition of key indicators can be helpful in solving a situation before it has the chance to manifest into an absolutely full blown disorder that might require professional help. Here are some helpful ideas for preventing burnout.

Pace Yourself

One of the most important things I had to master was how to create a healthy pace within my own work environment. I still struggle with this concept at times in my life. This would allow me the luxury of getting an objective completed without placing too much stress on my psyche. When you learn how to adhere to a healthy pace in your own life, this will do wonders for you.

If you think about this logically, it makes perfect sense. Imagine for a moment about how a long distance runner and a sprinter prepare for a competition. Both athletes compete in track events that require a different pace. If the two athletes did not have any idea about how far they would have to run they would have a difficult time becoming successful in each of their events. The pace that is used by the sprinter is certainly going to be different than the pace that is utilized by the long distance runner. Having a proper pace will ensure the two runners a better chance of success within their given categories of competition. The same logic can and should be applied when tackling projects in the workplace.

Allow Time for Rest & Relaxation

It is easy to let yourself become obsessed with a work project. I have done this many times in my own life. Having proper amounts of time set aside for periods of rest and relaxation will be quite helpful in keeping you fresh and recharged for when you do return to your place of business.

Rest and relaxation does not mean that you should just sit on the couch in front of the television for a couple of hours. Periods of rest and relaxation must have a definite quality built into them. Learn how to take vacations and get yourself away from daily routines. A change of scenery can also be helpful in getting you to become more relaxed. Even two or three day excursions to new destinations can be helpful in breaking the rut and boredom of the everyday grind. Remember that you work very hard for a living so it is important that you reward yourself during the year with multiple opportunities to get away from the workplace.

When you are on vacation do not take your cell phone or pager with you. If you take these items on a vacation, you are actually taking your work with you and you are not really removing yourself from the office. Make arrangements for someone to fill in for you at your business or shut the doors for a couple of days. Get your customers or your boss comfortable with the idea that you need to be sharp while working and in order to be at your best you need to rest and relax like anybody else. Do not be ashamed of taking time off from work so that you can go on a vacation. Practice good rest and relaxation habits and you will stay excited and fresh in the workplace for many years to come.

Spend Quality Time with Family

It is extremely important that you spend quality time with your spouse and children. I believe that a successful marriage is an important prerequisite for having a happy and successful business life. Keeping careful focus on the big picture of life and making sure that your domestic affairs are in order will go a long way in helping you to accomplish the various goals you set out to achieve.

It is not very realistic for people to believe that they will have success in running a business if in fact they constantly stumble in their attempts to have successful personal relationships. These two components of our lives are quite interrelated and will regularly impact one another. Individuals who become aware of the connection between the two components early in their careers are usually the people who are also successful in their business and work lives.

Celebrate the Goals You Achieve

In an earlier chapter I wrote about creating realistic goals. The point that I wanted to highlight in this heading is that many frustrations, as well as other emotional problems that are commonly observed as a result of life related stress, can be avoided altogether by simply making sure that the goals you set, in any area of your life, are kept realistic enough so you can achieve them.

Once you do achieve a goal do not be afraid to celebrate the accomplishment. As I continued to succeed in reaching my personal weight loss goals, I celebrated my accomplishments. I wrote about my program and charted my success. I also rewarded myself by doing something special for me. Be creative and treat yourself to a movie or buy a book that you have been meaning to read. Take the time to reward yourself for all the hard work that you have performed. Make sure that you also celebrate these accomplishments with your spouse and children who are your support team. Acknowledging the completion of one goal will absolutely help you to focus more clearly on the next objective on your list of priorities.

Have a Hobby

Having a hobby or an interest in a particular area that exists outside of your chosen profession is a great idea. People who devote all of their energy and spare time to the workplace are setting themselves up for problems.

I have always maintained a variety of hobbies which I like to devote time to. I am a chiropractor and college instructor by trade, but my professional resume does not make up my entire life. Although chiropractic is very important to me, it is by no means the only interest within my life. I have many hobbies that lie outside the lines of the chiropractic profession. These hobbies allow me to keep my professional life exciting. I do not become bored with my profession because I have learned to live with it harmoniously and I have learned to leave it on the shelf at times when I am doing something I enjoy which is outside of my professional life. I implore you to do the same in your own life.

The success I have recently enjoyed with my *waist away* program was facilitated by my ability to relearn how to think outside the box in certain situations. This ultimately allowed me to identify and correct some mild signs of work related burnout for a second time in my life. Although I could recognize conformity to conventionality as an epidemic problem within our own country, I could not, for some strange reason, identify the same exact problem within my own life.

We live, we experience and hopefully we are able to learn from our mistakes. I am grateful for the experience I have just gone through. I think that it will serve me well over the long haul and I can tell you for certain that it has motivated me beyond my wildest dreams to maintain my weight and health at optimum levels.

Even though I had written articles and books on the subjects of "thinking out of the box" and "job related burnout," I still fell victim to these mind traps. Human beings are not perfect and I certainly qualify as an example to drive home this point. In many instances, I could see in others what I was unable to see in me.

The actual benefit I received from my *waist away* program was twofold. I obviously benefited tremendously from the loss of weight on my body, but perhaps the most important benefit that came out of my campaign was restoring my own ability to recognize serious problems that had been affecting me for a long time.

Maintaining my Weight Loss
Results over a Lifetime

According to most healthcare experts, about 95% of the people who lose a substantial amount of weight are likely to gain all the weight back within a relatively short period of time. This statistic suggests that most people are failing miserably when battling the bulge. According to one source, *"... there is little support for the notion that diets lead to lasting weight loss or health benefits."* **Mann, T., Tomiyama, E., Westling, E., Samuels, B., Chatman, J. (2007) Medicare's Search for Effective Obesity Treatments: Diets Are Not the Answer -** *American Psychologist* **Vol. 62 No. 3, 220 – 233.**

I was determined to be one of the successful people who resided in the 5% column. I had worked too hard and for too long, designing my strategy, to have it simply pulled out from under me after I finally reached my goal. I think one of the reasons why so many people are not successful in maintaining their weight loss results is because they mistakenly believe that their work is over once they reach the weight they originally targeted. They do not create another set of realistic goals to maintain the level of success they achieved.

In my chiropractic practice there are many strategies I will employ in an effort to convince patients to maintain their spinal care over a lifetime and not just when it is their perception that a problem exists. This process of educating patients is for the healthcare consumer's benefit.

Through the years I have attempted to create finite time lines when designing plans of care for my patients so that they could gauge, in their own mind, where I was taking them and how long of a ride it was going to be. I would tell patients, in the initial stages of care, we had to stabilize their spines with a series of corrective care spinal adjustments. This would be followed by patient reevaluations after a specific period of time had passed. I would then explain to patients that once we reached a point where their spines were stable, we needed to set some maintenance goals so that the positive results we achieved would not deteriorate over time.

I needed to do the same thing in my weight loss program as I routinely did with the patients in my private office. I needed to create a maintenance program that would allow me to retain all of the benefits derived from the *waist away* program. This concept is not rocket science. It is however, paramount to the success of any weight loss strategy. If you only work hard at doing something for a short period of time, you are going to yield very limited results. There was no doubt in my mind that I would gain all of my weight back, with interest, if I decided to revert back to a sedentary lifestyle and I began to eat oversized portions of food once again.

My Maintenance Plan

When I designed the *waist away* program, I did so by implementing common sense strategies that have been utilized by people who have achieved and maintained weight loss results for many years. There were four basic principles in my program that I believe were the cornerstones of my success. They ultimately created the opportunities for me to achieve a successful weight loss result.

I knew from day one of my program that I would need to incorporate these four principles in my daily routine during the initial phase of losing weight as well as during the phase in which I would maintain my accomplishment. This is how I structured my maintenance program.

The Four Principles of Weight Loss Maintenance

1. I must continue to eat a healthy amount of quality kilocalories on a daily basis.

2. I must continue a daily walking program.

3. I must continue to weigh myself every day.

4. I must continue to receive regular chiropractic care.

These four principles would absolutely ensure that I would maintain my weight loss results indefinitely.

When I looked at the number of people in the United States that had successfully lost a significant amount of weight – *only to gain all or most of the weight back within a year* – I immediately realized that these folks were simply reverting back to their old lifestyles after reaching their goals.

Simple Mathematics

According to www.caloriesperhour.com, a 175 pound man burns the following kilocalories in a one hour period of time doing the following activities:

1 hour of walking 3.5 mph = 302 kcals burned

1 hour of sleeping = 71 kcals burned

1 hour of sitting   = 119 kcals burned

For the purpose of demonstrating to readers how this maintenance program works, I have created a completely hypothetical situation for your consideration. Let's pretend that I plan to walk 1 hour per day, sleep 8 hours per evening, and sit in a chair each day for 15 hours. I will perform these activities religiously for one year. If I was to adhere to this model every day for one entire year, I would hypothetically burn approximately 2,655 kilocalories each day. This means that I could eat and place into my body, on a daily basis, a total of the same amount of kilocalories that my metabolism was burning and I would neither gain nor lose any additional weight whatsoever.

Obviously, this is an unrealistic model as I can pretty much assure you that I do not plan to sit in a chair for 15 hours each day. I do however; plan to walk an hour each day and I do usually average about 8 hours of sleep each evening. If I bump my activity level up slightly to account for when I practice chiropractic in my office or the college where I instruct students, it would be safe to assume that the kilocalories I burned per day would increase to a range of about 2,700 – 3,200 kilocalories.

Applying the Four Principles

Utilizing the *four principles of weight loss maintenance* is not that difficult. I had been using these principles every single day for the past seven months. The only difference in my strategy during the maintenance phase of my program was to adjust the number of kilocalories being consumed from my diet so they were equal to the number of kilocalories being burned from my body's metabolism. This stuff is common sense and can be competently performed by any person who can operate a calculator, a scale, and can commit to a regular daily walking routine.

There is absolutely no reason why a person who engages in a realistic and well thought out weight loss program should ever have a problem reaching his or her goals. In addition, there is no reason why the same individual should ever gain back any of the weight that was initially lost.

The problem with most people in modern society is that they are not disciplined enough to commit to a walking routine or once they reach a goal they become complacent and develop apathetic attitudes about the major ingredients that support their continued good health.

I will attempt to maintain my accomplishment for the remainder of my life. There are three very important people counting on me to come through on my promise

– my wife, my daughter and me. When it comes right down to it you have to be motivated to do something as important as this campaign for selfish reasons. If you do not care about yourself, it is very unlikely that you will care about family members. I have to continue to remember that I will be of no use to my family if I die from an obesity related disease.

Through adequate nutrition, exercise, and chiropractic care, I have won the battle of the bulge. This is my story and I hope that readers have derived some sort of benefit from my experience.

Afterword

I believe that each person is very unique. I also believe it is unrealistic and quite ineffective to attempt to design a set menu that services the needs of everyone trying to achieve weight loss results. In this book I have listed some sample menus that I utilized in my *waist away* program (See Appendices A-E). I feel that readers should only use these sample diets as informational guides when putting together their own plans.

People have different food preferences. The various menus that I utilized to accomplish my goals might not be satisfactory for many readers. I want to convey in my writings that while it is important for you to select good and nutritious foods in your own menu, you must also remember to select the types of foods that you regularly enjoy eating.

Many people will struggle as they try to remove some of the unhealthy foods from their current diets. I remember how challenging it was when I gave up drinking soda. I was miserable and it took me several months to get over the cravings.

For those of you who consume large amounts of artificial sweeteners on a regular basis, I believe it would benefit you greatly to perform some independent research about these products to see if you still want to include them in your own diet. Access an Internet search engine and type in the words, *"The dangers associated with artificial sweeteners."* Obviously, readers will need to make up their own minds after reading the mounds of information that have been written about this very controversial subject. Nevertheless, it is important that you become cognizant of the fact that many professionals in the healthcare industry have written words of caution with regards to consuming artificial sweeteners.

If you are like most people, you probably enjoy going out to have a nice meal at a restaurant. When you construct your own diet, I would highly recommend that you create a list of the dining establishments you regularly frequent. Once you have secured your list, you can pick out the lower calorie dishes at a specific location. Many of your favorite restaurants will have the nutritional information you are looking for in a company brochure. If you cannot access the information directly from the source, you can always use the website www.dietfacts.com. This is a pretty nifty tool that can provide the consumer with nutritional information for just about every dish served in most of the major dining establishments throughout the United States. The website is also very user friendly.

You now need to take action and start planning your own *waist away* program. Be aggressive, and begin implementing your strategies for successful weight loss results today. **Remember to first consult your physician to make sure that you are healthy enough to take part in a weight loss program.**

I realize that it takes a lot of hard work to accomplish a specific goal, but any person can do what I did as long as he or she is willing to devote the time and the energy into a specific weight loss program. Good Luck!

Dr. John Reizer
Chiropractor

Appendix-A

My Typical 1,750 kilocalorie Diet:

BREAKFAST:

One Egg	90 kilocalories
One Cup of Non Fat Milk	90 kilocalories
One Cup of Watermelon	50 kilocalories
One Slice of Whole Wheat Bread	90 kilocalories
One Tablespoon of Grape Jelly	55 kilocalories

SNACK:

1 Granola Peanut Butter Bar	115 kilocalories

LUNCH:

2.5 oz of lean turkey meat	100 kilocalories
One Apple	80 kilocalories
½ of Pita pocket (whole wheat)	90 kilocalories
One Cup of spinach	14 kilocalories

SNACK:

1 Granola Peanut Butter Bar	115 kilocalories

DINNER:

2 cups of spaghetti (whole wheat)	300 kilocalories
3 oz of turkey	120 kilocalories
Raw onion slices (4)	10 kilocalories
Marinara Sauce 1 Cup	80 kilocalories
¼ cup of grated Parmesan Cheese	115 kilocalories

SNACK:

3 cups of Watermelon	150 kilocalories
1 apple	80 kilocalories

Appendix-B

My Typical 2,000 kilocalorie Diet:

BREAKFAST:

Three Cups of Bran Cereal	420 kilocalories
Two Cups of Non Fat Milk	180 kilocalories
One Banana	100 kilocalories

LUNCH:

4.0 oz of lean Roast Beef	150 kilocalories
One Apple	80 kilocalories
½ of Pita pocket (whole wheat)	90 kilocalories
One Cup of spinach14 kilocalories	

SNACK:

1 Apple	80 kilocalories

DINNER:

2 Personal sized Pizza Shells 7 inch	545 kilocalories
Marinara Sauce 2 Cups	160 kilocalories
¼ Cup of grated Parmesan Cheese	28 kilocalories

SNACK:

1 cup of Watermelon	50 kilocalories

Appendix-C

My Typical 2,700 kilocalorie Maintenance Diet:

BREAKFAST:

Three Cups of Bran Cereal	**420 kilocalories**
Two Cups of Non Fat Milk	**180 kilocalories**
One Banana	**100 kilocalories**

LUNCH:

Large Chef Salad	**600 kilocalories**
One Apple	**80 kilocalories**
One Dinner Roll (Whole Wheat)	**120 kilocalories**

SNACK:

1 Apple	**80 kilocalories**

DINNER:

2 Chicken Breasts	**300 kilocalories**
1 Baked Potato	**150 kilocalories**
¼ Cup of grated Parmesan Cheese	**110 kilocalories**
2 Cups of spinach	**28 kilocalories**
Ketchup for baked potato	**40 kilocalories**
Baby Carrots (raw)	**20 kilocalories**
1 Dinner Roll (Whole Wheat)	**120 kilocalories**

SNACK:

3 Cups of Watermelon	**150 kilocalories**
2 Bananas	**200 kilocalories**

Appendix – D

A 1,956 Kilocalorie Diet:

BREAKFAST:

1 bagel	180 kilocalories
1 tablespoon jelly	50 kilocalories
½ cup of orange juice	60 kilocalories

SNACK:

1 apple	50 kilocalories

LUNCH:

Salmon 3 oz (broiled)	150 kilocalories
One cup of clam chowder	80 kilocalories
Dinner salad with oil & vinegar	125 kilocalories
½ cup of brown rice	116 kilocalories
Water	0 kilocalories

SNACK:

1 pear	100 kilocalories

DINNER:

2 cups of spaghetti	300 kilocalories
1 cup of tomato sauce	80 kilocalories
¼ cup of grated Parmesan Cheese	110 kilocalories
2 cups of spinach	28 kilocalories
2 cups of mixed vegetables	232 kilocalories
Dinner salad (oil & vinegar)	125 kilocalories
1 dinner roll (whole wheat)	120 kilocalories

SNACK:

12 grapes	50 kilocalories

Appendix – E

A 1,728 Kilocalorie Diet:

BREAKFAST:

1 slice of whole wheat bread	120 kilocalories
1 scrambled egg	90 kilocalories
½ cup of apple juice	60 kilocalories

SNACK:

1 orange	65 kilocalories

LUNCH:

Chicken 3 oz (broiled)	140 kilocalories
1 spinach wrap	110 kilocalories
Dinner salad with oil & vinegar	125 kilocalories
Mustard	5 kilocalories
Water	0 kilocalories

SNACK:

1 apple	80 kilocalories

DINNER:

1 sirloin steak (7 0z)	420 kilocalories
1 baked potato	150 kilocalories
2 cups of spinach	28 kilocalories
1 small salad (oil & vinegar)	125 kilocalories
1 dinner roll (whole wheat)	120 kilocalories
Ketchup (for potato)	40 kilocalories

SNACK:

1 cup of watermelon	50 kilocalories

Dr. John Reizer

Update – June, 2010

On August 31, 2007 I officially attained my original weight loss goal of 175 pounds. It was only a short time after this date that I completed work on the "Waist Away" book. What would happen to my body after August 31, 2007 was a major concern in my life at that time. Perhaps the most important personal goal that I would ever set was designing my very own foolproof plan that would ultimately ensure that I maintained my successful weight loss results indefinitely.

From the onset of my journey, I decided that I never wanted to live again in a body that was overweight or obese. This had been a horrible experience and it was territory that I had left behind and had absolutely no desire to revisit in the future.

It is now June 8, 2010 (I am 47 years old) and as I sit in my home office, I am happy and proud to report that I have continued to follow my program.

As the months and years have passed, I continued to maintain my weight loss results. I eventually leveled off at a weight of 162 pounds and have maintained that same weight since the inception of my program back in January, 2007.

I continue to eat a very healthy diet and I never walk around hungry. I am actually eating more food than ever before and it does not matter whether I am on vacation, eating at a restaurant, or dining in the comfort of my home. The point I am trying to make is that I have adapted very well to my new lifestyle. I have recalibrated my brain to recognize the difference between eating healthy and unhealthy foods. I have also trained my body to respond positively when I take part in healthy sessions of exercise. I have completely embraced the *Waist Away Program* and it has absolutely changed and saved my life at the same time.

In one year I dropped **83 pounds**, and I continue to feel great. I honestly believe that I am the healthiest I have ever been in my entire life. When I look at pictures of me from a few years ago compared to pictures of me now, it is hard for me to believe that I am looking at the same person.

Waist Away

Once again, I want to encourage and challenge my readers to set and attain similar weight loss goals for themselves. This is an opportunity for you to make an investment in your health and well being. I know for certain that this is an investment that will absolutely pay you and your family dividends for many years to come.

Dr. John Reizer

Chiropractor

www.ingramcontent.com/pod-product-compliançe
Lightning Source LLC
Chambersburg PA
CBHW051349280526
45784CB00007B/2888